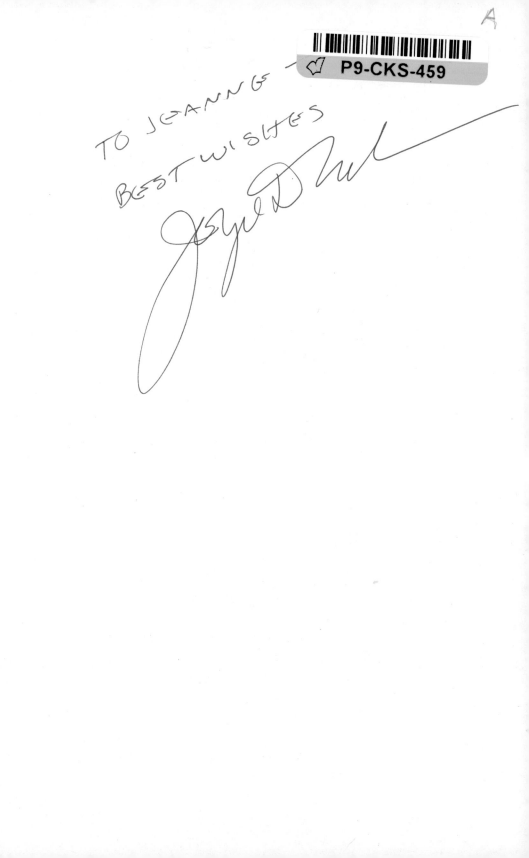

TO JOANNG —

BEST WISHES

What Your Doctor *Can't* Tell You About

COSMETIC SURGERY

Other Books by the Author

Now That You've Lost It

Maximize Your Body Potential

Taking Charge of Your Smoking

Taking Charge of Your Weight and Well-Being
(with Linda Ormiston)

What Your Doctor *Can't* Tell You About

COSMETIC SURGERY

JOYCE D. NASH, PH.D.

NEW HARBINGER PUBLICATIONS, INC.

Publisher's Note

This publication is designed to provide accurate and authoritative information in regard to the subject matter covered. It is sold with the understanding that the publisher is not engaged in rendering pyschological, financial, legal, or other professional services. If expert assistance or counseling is needed, the services of a competent professional should be sought.

Cover design and illustration by Lightbourne Images © 1995.
Text design by Tracy Marie Powell.
Photos in this book were supplied by Archive Photos.

Distributed in U.S.A. primarily by Publishers Group West; in Canada by Raincoast Books; in Great Britain by Airlift Book Company, Ltd.; in South Africa by Real Books, Ltd.; in Australia by Boobook; in New Zealand by Tandem Press.

Library of Congress Catalog Card Number: 95-69485

ISBN 1-57224-033-4 hardcover
ISBN 1-57224-032-6 paperback

First printing 1995, 5,000 copies

Contents

Acknowledgments

Acknowledgements are gratefully extended to those who shared their stories and experiences of cosmetic surgery and in many cases completed questionnaires; to friends and colleagues who read early drafts and offered valuable suggestions—Sylvia Dostal, Geri Gunkelberger, Cathy Latta, Judy Ross, Claudia Siegel, and Pamela Swales; to David White, M.D., who provided technical assistance with the information on plastic surgery; to Matt McKay of New Harbinger Publications, who saw the value of this work; to Patrick Fanning, Kirk Johnson, Gayle Zanca, and Tracy Powell, who are largely responsible for bringing it to publication; to Lauren Dockett, who handled publicity and promotions for the book; to Virginia Lewis, who supported me through my own cosmetic surgery experience; and to my husband, Morgan White, for his patience and support of my work on this project.

Introduction

"Come now! Let me dress you like your sisters!" She put a wreath of white lilies in her hair, but every petal of the flowers was half a pearl; and the old lady put eight oysters on the Princess's tail, to show her high rank.

"But it hurts!" said the little mermaid.

"Yes, but one must suffer to be beautiful," said the old lady . . .

—The Little Mermaid
by Hans Christian Andersen

Several months after my face-lift surgery, I began to reflect on the experience. I am trained as a clinical psychologist. How could I have been so unprepared for the physical and emotional trauma it brought? Had I missed something the doctor said? I had read the pamphlets I was given and watched a video beforehand in the doctor's office. I had leafed through his album of former patients. The doctor and staff answered the questions I asked. I even talked to a former patient of my doctor about her experience with the same operation. She had let me see pictures of herself before surgery and several months after. The results of my surgery were dramatic and technically excellent. In fact, my doctor requested permission to put my before-and-after photos in a textbook illustrating what cosmetic surgery can accomplish. Still, I was not prepared for the initial pain, depression, and impact on my body image that cosmetic surgery brought. Nor was I prepared for the enduring physical changes, including tightness, skin discoloration, and change in sensation. Were my reactions unusual, or do others have similar experiences? These questions prompted me to begin my inquiry into the psychology of cosmetic surgery, and ultimately led to the writing of this book.

Nothing the doctor says fully prepares you for the physical and psychological trauma of cosmetic surgery. Almost always, the pain is underestimated. Pamphlets, brochures, and books that claim the pain is "easily controlled by medications" understate the reality, at least for some procedures. Medication can take the edge off pain, but it cannot eliminate it altogether. There is unforeseen pain, unfamiliar pain. Pain, together with the inevitable bruising, swelling, general discomfort, and interruption of daily routine that accompanies cosmetic surgery, can trigger psychological trauma. Reactions can range from a vague sense of loss to full-fledged grief, anger, and depression. A temporary identity disturbance can occur—and even psychosis in rare instances. Sometimes initial euphoria gives way to a downward emotional slide. Most people are pleased with the outcome of cosmetic surgery, but, in spite of sometimes numerous consultations with doctors, few people comprehend what they will have to endure for the promise of enhanced beauty.

In 1992 alone, more than 1.5 million Americans underwent plastic surgery, of which 395,000 had elective cosmetic procedures. (Cosmetic surgery is a subset of plastic surgery with the purpose of altering appearance so patients will feel better about themselves.) Although patients are informed about the technical aspects of surgery and its results, a 1992 study contends that surgeons tend to minimize the pain, trauma, and temporary disfigurement involved.[1] According to this research, the level of post-operative trauma and distress, as observed by nurses attending cosmetic surgery patients, is much greater than surgeons are aware or patients are led to expect. A large majority of patients in this study experienced post-operative physical trauma and significant emotional distress during the months following surgery. Patients need to be better informed about what to expect during recovery, and better prepared to deal with the distress that even a desired change in appearance can bring.

An earlier study of 599 patients undergoing various cosmetic and plastic surgery procedures found that 32 percent showed transient psychological effects soon after surgery, mainly anxiety and depression.[2] The researchers felt these were "normal" reactions to swelling, hematoma, and the physical trauma of surgery. Still other reports put the rate of post-operative anxiety or depression at 55 percent. In a study of 50 women undergoing face-lift surgery, 24 percent suffered a period of depression lasting days, and 30 percent developed a depression that lasted two to three weeks.[3] For some, post-operative depression lasts months and even years.

Other psychological reactions are perhaps less frequent but nonetheless disturbing. Initial reactions upon recovering from the anesthesia are often fear, grief, and even anger. That first look in the mirror is usually a shock. Breast surgery patients may have persistent nightmares of having deformed breasts long after surgery, even though their "new" breasts are fine. Nose reshaping has led to the experience of loss of identity and even, in rare cases, psychotic decompensation (the breakdown of ability to cope with the ordinary demands of life, leading to an exacerbation of or triggering a mental disorder). All of this can happen despite the fact that these patients had *objectively good* results, that is, results that all but the patient agree are good.

Research shows that cosmetic surgery generally brings psychological improvement for most patients. But there is more than meets the eye to cosmetic surgery. Although patient satisfaction tends to be high, adverse psychological reactions, as well as physical trauma, are more common than is generally understood. Doctors want their patients to be aware of the risks of cosmetic surgery, as well as its benefits, but this is often difficult if not impossible to achieve.

Surgeons acknowledge the difficulty of fully informing prospective patients. They provide one or more consultations to assess the patient's prospects and appropriateness for surgery, and they attempt to explain the risks and benefits involved. Often such consultations are accompanied by viewing a videotape on cosmetic surgery or seeing possible changes through computer imaging. Sometimes photo albums of before-and-after pictures are available, although surgeons are sensitive to maintaining patient confidentiality and may not have such pictures to show. If they do, the viewer should be aware that only the best results are likely to be exhibited, despite the fact that any practicing surgeon inevitably has had some less-than-satisfactory outcomes. Another reason surgeons may not want to show before-and-after pictures is that by doing so there may be an implied guarantee of results that could carry increased liability for the surgeon. Also there are brochures on virtually every procedure, created by professional organizations and purchased by doctors for distribution to potential patients. A number of plastic surgeons or their representatives have also written books on cosmetic surgery. Most of these focus on the technical details of various operations from the surgeon's perspective.

What Your Doctor Can't *Tell You About Cosmetic Surgery* is the first book to describe the *patient's experience* and tell the reader what surgeons *cannot* tell their patients—that is, what it is really like to undergo cosmetic surgery. Unlike others, this book describes motivations and expectations, who seeks surgery and why, patient satisfaction and dissatisfaction with various operations, how to prepare for surgery and recovery, the impact of surgery on body image, social taboos and the reactions of spouses and significant others, the doctor/patient relationship, and the factors that determine whether a patient is likely to experience the outcome as good or bad. This book attempts to redress the imbalance of information prospective patients get about cosmetic surgery. It is intended to be an informative self-help book that provides a realistic picture of the range of emotions and physical experiences that can occur days, months, and even years after obtaining cosmetic surgery. Readers should be better able to make an informed decision about such surgery.

The intent is not to disparage cosmetic surgery. The focus is not on horror stories of mutilation resulting from cosmetic surgery, although some accounts of patients who were unhappy with their results are included. Nor is this a sales pitch for cosmetic surgery. The book does not get into the technical details of various operations or offer suggestions on how to find a surgeon. Rather, my aim is to provide a better understanding of the psychological forces that influence the motivation for surgery, the decision-making process, and the recovery period that follows surgery. In addition, I detail the social and cultural influences at work at every stage. As a result, readers should be better able to make informed decisions about whether to proceed with cosmetic surgery, and if they do, to prepare adequately for it.

Patients undergoing any type of surgery benefit by becoming psychologically prepared. Studies have found that when patients are adequately prepared, they experience less pain, require less pain medication, recuperate faster with fewer complications, suffer less psychological distress, and show greater satisfaction with the outcome.[4] Planning, problem solving, and supportive attitudes prior to surgery can help patients cope more effectively. Books and manuals aimed at helping patients prepare for surgery of any type are only now beginning to be written. This book is the first to prepare the reader psychologically for cosmetic surgery.

The psychology of cosmetic surgery is still young and as yet poorly understood. Early research was heavily influenced by surgeons and psychiatrists trying to integrate somatic and psychological aspects in the understanding and treatment of those requesting cosmetic procedures. Initial research consisted mostly of case reports of patients evaluated from a psychoanalytic point of view and emphasizing individual dynamics. The possibility of healthy motivation for cosmetic surgery was entirely overlooked, and cultural and social influences were neglected. Too much emphasis was put on personality factors and individual psychopathology. The motivation for cosmetic surgery was assumed to be a sign of "neurosis," which is defined as a mental disorder in which the person is in touch with reality, but has symptoms such as anxiety, depression, phobias, compulsions, and dissociation. (These symptoms are distressing or unacceptable to the "neurotic" person, but his behavior is within normal social limits. By contrast, "psychosis" involves the inability to distinguish reality from fantasy and involves impaired ability to accurately understand or construe the world outside the self.) The presumption was that the underlying conflict was best treated with psychotherapy to avoid a "mere" symptom cure. Getting patients to see a psychiatrist, however, proved difficult; patients wanted surgery, not therapy.

Subsequent research tried to assess groups of patients more objectively, using questionnaires and standardized psychological tests administered before and after surgical procedures. Patient satisfaction became an important focus of study. Results indicated that patients were surprisingly satisfied with the results of surgery. This research suggested that a statistically significant number of patients showed a reduction in pre-existing psychiatric symptoms and an overall improvement in psychological well-being. Indeed, cosmetic surgery itself turned out to be a kind of psychotherapy. As a group, cosmetic surgery patients were found to be "normal," or at least not as severely psychologically disturbed as had been thought formerly. Satisfaction with the outcome of surgery was not significantly correlated with individual factors such as personality, psychopathology, or motivation. However, this research applied to groups, rather than to individuals, and it was not possible to say that these findings applied to any given patient.

As the influence of psychoanalytic thinking about cosmetic surgery patients began to wane, the psychology of cosmetic surgery began to be seen in a different light. No simple cause-and-effect relationship explains why people seek cosmetic surgery or how they react to it. Rather, an interdependent network of personal, social, and cultural factors contribute in a circular, rather than a linear, fashion. A much broader array of forces are now seen as influencing patient behavior and attitude. These are personal factors that include beliefs, motivations, expectations, and thinking styles, as well as character traits. All of these influence an individual's decision to have surgery. Rather than hidden conflicts, the particular coping skills and abilities of a prospective patient are emerging as particularly important for a good recovery. A person's significant others, peer group, professional situation—even the choice of a particular surgeon—influence both the choice to have surgery and the recovery process. Personal and social factors operate in a cultural context that becomes an overarching influence. Pressure to conform to socially defined ideals of beauty cannot be ignored as an important influence, and admonitions to ignore such pressure and "accept yourself as you are" can fall on deaf ears.

Clearly, the primary audience for this book are those who may be thinking about obtaining cosmetic surgery. It is also intended for their friends and loved ones, because social influences are important in both the decision to have surgery and in the recovery process. Another audience, however, is plastic surgeons, their staff, and surgical nurses. Often doctors are not completely aware of the psychological trauma that their patients can experience, partly because patients are reluctant to tell them. They often want to be "good patients" and to please the doctor. If issues are raised, it is often to the doctor's nurse, who may or may not give much weight to the patient's concerns. This book can help sensitize doctors, nurses, and support staff to the often hidden psychological and physical experiences of their patients. Finally, this book is appropriate for psychiatrists, psychologists, and other mental health professionals who have a particular interest in health psychology, body image, or women's issues.

I am uniquely qualified to write this book. I am a clinical psychologist, and in 1991 I underwent a radical face-lift procedure. Although the outcome was excellent, I had a difficult recovery. I experienced firsthand the powerful psychological force that feelings about the body can have on the mind. Despite being a psychologist and having knowledge of human emotions and behavior, nothing in my training or in consultations with my surgeon.prepared me for the pain and emotional impact of this surgery.

In this book, I lead the reader through the stages of the cosmetic surgery experience: the first stirrings of motivation, the decision-making process, the commitment to proceed, the operating room, and then recovery. At each stage of the process, the underlying psychological forces are described. Throughout, I offer information and suggestions to help prospective patients decide whether to proceed with cosmetic surgery, as well as advice on how to better prepare themselves, should they decide to go ahead.

The actual experiences of cosmetic surgery patients illustrate the scientific concepts that have emerged from research on the psychological aspects of cosmetic surgery. In detail I describe my own experience, as well as that of two other cosmetic surgery patients, Jackie, who underwent a breast lift and augmentation, and Paulette, who had a nose reshaping. In addition to these three detailed patient experiences, sketches of other patients are included. Except for the author, the names and identifying information of the other patients have been changed. Although this book is not intended to be a scholarly text, citations of relevant research are given in case the reader wants to further explore a particular issue.

Personal interviews and responses to a questionnaire provided many of the experiences that I describe. For the most part, the stories told are about people who have had objectively good results and are pleased with the outcome. The book concludes with practical advice from former patients and with a discussion of how therapy can be helpful as an adjunct, or alternative, to surgery.

For the most part, I use "he" when referring to surgeons and "she" when referring to patients. There are, of course, female surgeons and male patients. I use these pronouns in this way because most plastic surgeons (about 90 percent) are male, and most patients (about 86 percent) are female, and because it is cumbersome to use the linked, but admittedly, more egalitarian "he and she" convention. I ask the reader's forbearance in this matter.

Chapter 1 begins with an explanation of why doctors have difficulty informing patients about the risks, complications, and recovery process involved in cosmetic surgery. Often prospective patients don't get the information they need to make a considered decision about cosmetic surgery or to prepare adequately.

Chapter 2 focuses on the personal impact of a perceived physical imperfection and the social importance of appearance. Beauty is in "the eye of the beholder," and how one views oneself is more important than how others perceive a possible shortcoming. Beauty has high currency in American society, especially for women, and is very relevant to the motivation for cosmetic surgery.

Various explanations for why people seek cosmetic surgery have been offered by both the psychiatric community and by feminists. Chapter 3 explores these explanations, as well as the research findings on motivation and patient expectations for cosmetic surgery. In addition to offering an alternative, "healthy motivation" explanation, this chapter helps readers decide if they are good candidates for cosmetic surgery.

Chapter 4 presents a brief account of each of the main cosmetic surgery procedures and the psychological factors associated with them. Some operations produce more dramatic change than others. As a result, some operations are more likely to be associated with psychological trauma.

Women, as well as men, teens, children, the elderly, ethnic minorities, and others seek cosmetic surgery. Chapter 5 considers the psychological factors involved in those who seek certain types of surgery.

Chapter 6 focuses on the process of deciding whether to proceed with surgery and on the preparation needed to increase the chances of a good result. This chapter discusses what goes on in the consultation with a plastic surgeon and how patients typically prepare for surgery.

The early recovery period—the time immediately after surgery and extending for two to three months—is when physical trauma, including pain, swelling, and bruising, is most acute. This is also the time when psychological reactions such as depression, remorse, anger, and grief are likely to be apparent. In detailing these reactions from the perspective of actual patients, Chapter 7 tells the readers what the doctor can't tell them.

Chapter 8 is an important follow-on to the preceding chapter, because it describes the impact of cosmetic surgery on self-concept and body image—the mental and psychological picture a person holds of him- or herself. Each part of the body has symbolic meanings that are relevant to body image. In this chapter, readers have an opportunity to assess their own body image.

In Chapter 9, the social influences at each step of the way take center stage. Sources of social taboos related to cosmetic surgery are discussed. Reactions of friends and loved ones to the idea or reality of cosmetic surgery, before, during, and after, are considered. This chapter raises the question, Who do you tell and when do you tell them?

Chapter 10 focuses on patient satisfaction with results and the need to come to terms with post-operative complications and unmet expectations. Cosmetic surgery involves trade-offs that often are not apparent in the initial stages of thinking about surgery and then deciding to go ahead with it. This chapter suggests that the notion of "complete recovery" is relative. Warning signs are identified that can signal possible unfavorable reactions to cosmetic surgery.

Sometimes things do go wrong. Chapter 11 considers what can cause patient dissatisfaction, what makes things go wrong, and the importance of the doctor-patient relationship. Although objectively bad results are unusual, some patients are dissatisfied with the way they look, even though others see no problem. In rare cases, results are objectively bad. This chapter also discusses the psychiatrically impaired patient and the relationship of emotional disturbance to dissatisfaction with results.

Even though patients seeking cosmetic procedures want surgery, not therapy, there are times when a psychiatric consultation or even therapy is appropriate. Chapter 12 discusses the indications for and benefits of therapy, and how coping is related to outcome.

Who better to offer insight and advice about cosmetic surgery than those who have had it? Chapter 13 offers the thoughts and suggestions of those who have gone before. Finally, in the epilogue, I offer my answer to the question so many have asked, "Would you do it again?"

1

Why Your Doctor
Can't Tell You

Kathy was in the waiting room of the plastic surgeon's office when she overheard the doctor's receptionist on the telephone.

"Why, there's little pain involved at all. You'll be back to work in a few days." It sounded so casual and easy, as if it warranted about as much thought as getting a facial or a new hairdo.

When patients are not fully aware of the physical and psychological risks and ramifications of cosmetic surgery, they can suffer considerable pain, emotional distress, financial cost, interference with life choices, and a loss of trust in health care professionals. Merilyn Evans, a research fellow at the Centre for Research in Public Health and Nursing at La Trobe University, Melbourne, Australia, argues that patients need more information so that they can make informed decisions. Evans provides the following account of a 27-year-old Australian woman who had a breast augmentation but did not get adequate information beforehand. Although this is an actual patient's account of her experience, it is not typical of a consultation, nor was it properly done. Information was misrepresented to this patient and claims were made that were inappropriate and misleading. It is not possible to tell from this account whether the surgeon was indeed qualified to perform plastic surgery. Chapter 6 discusses how to assess a surgeon's credentials in order to avoid this sort of disaster.

I had no idea that things could go wrong. For years everything I'd read was always positive—that cosmetic operations had been perfected and everything is fine. I've been flat chested since my teens, and I'd been rowing to try and increase my bust line. I couldn't understand why my mother and two sisters had boobs and I didn't. I used to pad my bra, like all young kids do, and then I had to keep doing it when it became obvious that I wasn't going to get any bigger. Then as I got older I used to get ribbed a lot—not usually with partners but other people. It was always tits, tits, tits everywhere you looked, especially when you went swimming. All the ads used to make me feel inadequate.

Then on the spur of the moment I decided to have the operation. It was just after a broken relationship and I had been saving up to go overseas. That was in December 1989 and I heard about it from another woman who'd had it done. I talked to her about it and she said, "It's great, you'll feel like a million dollars." We had a couple of days together and she told of her experience. All she had was a tiny bit of bruising and she was told to massage her breasts. I didn't need a referral; I just went straight to the same doctor and he sort of poked at me and said, "No, you haven't got much there have you? Yes, we can do something for you," and he plopped an implant into my hand. I asked him to tell me of any risks and he said there were three things I should know: that I would not have any scarring because he would cut around the nipple line and it would fade (which it has); that bleeding hardly ever happens; and that he had never had an infection occur. About 1 out of 100 people get hardening in one or both breasts. [This is a misstatement; the proportion of patients who experience hardening in one or both breasts is closer to 30 percent.] He really conveyed that there were never any problems, and that it was just like getting a tooth out. I thought I may as well get it done straight away. Mum thought I should wait a bit, but I decided to have it done in the Christmas holidays.

I knew something was wrong the moment they took the bandages off. I looked just like an inflated Barbie doll. The right breast was very hard, the left a bit softer but it still felt so tight and the pressure was incredible on both sides. I had a couple of plasters on around the nipples and they were sort of pointing downwards. I asked for a mirror and when I saw what I looked like I just burst into tears.

I had told him I didn't want to be too big; I just wanted my body to be a bit more balanced. All he said was that the implants would be about 250 milliliters, which just makes you think of milk bottles, doesn't it? I had asked him about breast-feeding and he had said it would not be a problem, but why have I lost sensation in my nipples? Sometimes now they feel so cold they could have come out of an icebox. Oh, he did take out a black marking pen and drew lines all over my chest. He said, "This is what we do," but it was a bit technical and didn't tell me anything really.

I went back three times to see another doctor (my own surgeon was away due to the holiday period) because I was worried about bruising from neck to groin. I knew it was not right, but he was a bit blasé and said, "I really think you're overreacting to this. There's a bit of scar tissue there and it will settle down in about six months." He either lied to me or he was really wet behind the ears. None of the staff explained anything after the operation—not the massage or lifting. I was lying down flat because of the bandages, and they sort of dragged me up in the bed by the armpits because I could hardly move myself. They were rough and it hurt and they really made me feel vain and neurotic.

The whole thing cost me heaps. I had to pay the surgeon $1,200 up front and an extra $700 or $800 for the implants. He told me the anesthesiologist and the hospital costs would be rebateable but they were not. It probably cost me $5,000 all up. And now I've got to start saving to get whatever has happened to me fixed. I hope I won't be paying for this for the rest of my life.[1]

Scheduling a consultation appointment with a surgeon is usually the first step for actually initiating cosmetic surgery. Both on the phone and when the patient enters the office, the staff are cordial and enthusiastic. Usually the prospective patient has several questions uppermost on her mind: What can be done? Can I afford it? Is this the doctor I want to have do it?

Most people would agree that every patient has the right to decide for or against a medical treatment, and that in order to do this, the patient must understand what the recommended procedure is, its purpose, the risks and complications, as well as the benefits and alternatives. John and Marcia Goin, a plastic surgeon and psychiatrist respectively, in their 1981 textbook *Changing the Body: Psychological Effects of Plastic Surgery*, argue that informed consent is a great idea but one that "simply doesn't work." This is partly because doctors don't always provide what is necessary for meaningful consent, and partly because prospective patients often are not able to comprehend the information the doctor gives them.

Informed Consent

A few doctors reportedly have tried to justify giving minimal information to patients, arguing that medical aspects and health care are their domain and that they can exercise their discretion in disclosing risks.[2] Actually, doctors are legally and ethically bound to involve patients in the decision to proceed with cosmetic surgery. Getting the patient's agreement and signature on a consent form is not enough, however. Valid informed consent means that the patient has been provided with adequate information and comprehends this information. Risks and potential harm, as well as benefits, must be communicated.

Legally, doctors are not required to discuss at length every conceivable complication that might occur, nor is it necessary to disclose "slight" risks from commonplace procedures. For example, discussing the possibility of developing a rash in reaction to the application of a dressing is not necessary, even if that rash might be painful. A California Supreme Court ruled that doctors need to address risk of serious injury or death, as well as risks related to recuperation.

Unfortunately, it is possible to "inform" without imparting much information. Increasingly, plastic surgeons are using both print and broadcast media to convey the easy availability and affordability of cosmetic surgery. Professionally developed marketing materials further promote the benefits while often downplaying complications. Nurses and staff in the doctor's office present a positive view of results and recovery, with little mention of difficulties patients can suffer. In the consultation with a prospective patient, the surgeon has his own agenda. One of his objectives is to assess the appropriateness of the person before him for surgery. In addition to discussing any serious risks, he wants to provide reassurance, reduce anxiety, and facilitate her proceeding with surgery if she is a good candidate. To demonstrate that the consent session has taken place, the doctor requests that the patient sign an informed consent form. Most surgeons augment verbal information with brochures and written information and perhaps videotape instruction or computer imaging.

Doctors try, but they *can't* tell potential patients everything they need to know about cosmetic surgery. Time is limited for consultations, and most doctors are busy assessing whether a person is appropriate for surgery. When talking to a prospective patient, a surgeon tends to emphasize the technical aspects of surgery and its results, while minimizing the pain and trauma involved. Often what is omitted during the consultation is more significant than what is said. In some cases, patients don't want to know about risks and complications, and some doctors include a section on their informed consent forms for patients to sign indicating they don't want to know and don't want to discuss complications. Furthermore, doctors often aren't fully aware of what patients go through. Patients rarely reveal their emotional reactions to their surgeons, and research on this topic is only beginning to tell the whole story.

Patients' Reactions to Pre-Operative Information

Cosmetic surgery patients have a great deal of difficulty comprehending information the doctor provides about the risks and complications of a proposed operation. By the time a patient decides to go for a consultation, she is already thinking more about the pros than the cons. Often a patient's mind is largely made up before the consultation, and her attention is focused on getting support for her decision, deciding if she trusts this particular doctor, and thinking about how she can afford the surgery, which is rarely covered by insurance.

Often patients remember only what they want to remember.[3] In some cases, patients are unwilling to acknowledge the possibility of post-operative complications, even when they are given this information in written form.[4] Even when warned that they will be asked to recall the information, patients can recall only about 35 percent of information given them.[5] Many prospective patients want to believe that cosmetic surgery is virtually risk-free. Psychologically, patients appear to engage in denial and repression to avoid unpleasant facts about the operations. In one study of 20 face-lift patients, 10 flatly denied that a complication could happen to them or admitted to deliberately putting the possibility out of mind.[6] Of these 20 patients, only 3 remembered three of the ten complications the doctor mentioned. Eight recalled one of the complications, and 9 were unable or unwilling to remember any complications told to them. In a few cases, patients felt they were immune to suffering any complications because they "healed well," or meditated, or took mega-doses of vitamins. Others believed that by having the "right" doctor they could eliminate risks. Only 10 percent of these patients experienced any fear of complications.

Whether it is cosmetic surgery or some other kind of treatment, patients frequently misunderstand or get wrong ideas about what they were told of the operation. Fully two-thirds of those who volunteered to participate in a study of a new anti-inflammatory drug forgot information about the most important complication.[7] Cardiac surgery patients who had been hospitalized for various procedures many times before (and thus could be expected to be familiar with procedures for their condition) were given structured, informed consent interviews that were also tape-recorded.[8] Subsequent interviews were conducted with patients who were convalescing normally to determine what patients remembered from the lengthy, pre-operative informed consent session. Several patients denied *any recollection whatever* of the previous interview. Only 10 percent recalled information of potential complications without prompting. Even with prompting only 23 percent recalled information on complications.

As if forgetting and misunderstanding weren't bad enough, 65 percent of patients sometimes "bring in their own facts." This erroneous information may have been acquired originally from another source, such as the media, another doctor, or another person. Self-assured individuals in particular tend to be convinced of their own facts and recollections, even if these are incorrect. In one study, several patients asserted that their informed consent interviews were very brief, even though the evidence indicated otherwise.

Some patients are better able than others to comprehend information given to them about risks and complications. Better educated patients, those having more than just a high school degree, understood and remembered more than those with a high school education or less. Patients who admitted to being nervous during the informed consent interview retained about 48 percent of what they heard, whereas calm patients remembered 30 percent. When information is given in written form, sicker patients remember less, perhaps because they are less careful in reading written consent information. Careful readers recalled significantly more than those who read only parts of the information given.

In summary, those who are most likely to comprehend the information necessary to make an informed decision are better educated and careful readers, anxious enough to stimulate attention (but not overanxious), and able to attend to the information given. Even so, denial and repression are significant obstacles to informing potential patients, and doctors protect themselves by documenting the details of informed consent, and by having the patient sign a form that says the informed consent interview took place.

Despite the doctor's best efforts, patients often don't get the information they need. When this happens, the patient's ability to make an informed decision is reduced. She is less able to prepare appropriately for surgery because she doesn't understand what to expect. When unexpected pain or complications appear, the doctor-patient relationship may suffer.

Informed Decision Making

Informed consent requires clear, two-way communication between doctor and patient. It involves more than just the provision of information about the risks and benefits of cosmetic surgery. As articulated by the President's Commission for the Study of Ethical Problems in Medicine and Biomedical and Behavioral Research, informed consent is the process of patient and doctor collaborating in a shared decision-making process that combines their unique perspectives and values to decide what treatment is in the patient's best interest. This process may at times involve getting a psychiatric consultation.

Prospective cosmetic surgery patients need to consider carefully the sort of questions that ought to be asked of the surgeon they consult. (See Chapter 6 for a detailed discussion of these issues.) Careful consideration should be given to his background and training, especially his experience in performing the particular operation under consideration. Bad results are often attributable to surgeons who have little or no specific training and little experience in cosmetic surgery procedures. A surgeon who is too eager to get the patient scheduled for surgery or who offers a bargain basement fee should be regarded with suspicion. The prospective patient should expect the surgeon to ask about her expectations for surgery, her motivation, and how long she has been concerned with the perceived defect in appearance. The doctor who does not ask such questions is not doing an adequate evaluation. Doctors and patients together need to ask: "Is the contemplated operation really necessary?

Is there a real choice? What other choices exist? Do we both know and understand the probable and possible outcomes—good and bad?"[9]

Summary

Doctors want their patients to be informed and to understand what the surgery they are considering implies. Unfortunately, this goal is harder to accomplish than it would appear. Patients often attend selectively to information that supports their wish to improve their appearance, and they tend to screen out information about risks or post-operative complications. Likewise, surgeons are generally more comfortable with the technical details than with the emotional aspects of the decision to proceed with cosmetic surgery. Patients give their consent for the operation by signing a form indicating that they understand the risks involved. Although this document may provide some legal protection to the doctor, the "informed consent" it refers to does not help the patient, either to make an informed decision, or to prepare adequately for the rigors of recovery. The process of making a truly informed decision begins *before* going for the first consultation. It begins by gathering information from other sources, such as by talking to those who have had cosmetic surgery and reading reliable published information on the procedure of interest, and then involving the surgeon and perhaps other professionals in the decision.

Some Questions to Ask Yourself

1. Can I describe what feature I am dissatisfied with and why, and what I want from cosmetic surgery?

2. Am I prepared to take longer to recuperate, including staying out of sight if necessary, than the doctor predicts?

3. Am I prepared to go through fear, regret, guilt, and anxiety in the first few hours or days after surgery, trusting these feelings will pass?

4. Am I prepared to suffer feeling sad, down, blue, tearful, and depressed for several weeks or even months, and if necessary seek professional help in this regard?

5. Am I prepared to look and feel worse before I look and feel better?

6. Am I prepared to tolerate numbness, changed skin sensitivity, tightness and pulling, skin discoloration, and other unforeseen "minor" complications—some of which may be permanent?

7. Am I prepared for my friends and loved ones to be upset, frightened, distant, unsupportive, or critical during the early recovery period and perhaps at other times?

8. Who will I blame if something goes wrong?

2

Eye of the Beholder

"A sack of broken eggs. That's what they look like." No matter that her friends thought her breasts looked just fine; Jackie was dissatisfied.

Chris, age 17, always wore big, baggy shirts to cover up her very large breasts. They were a source of painful attention when men openly admired her well-endowed chest.

"My nose looks too Jewish." Paul was convinced he would do better in his sales career if only his nose looked different. Paul's father bristled at the idea of cosmetic surgery. "It's our family nose. It was good enough for my father. It's good enough for me. It should be good enough for you. It suits us."

Recent years have witnessed an increasing demand for cosmetic surgery. This is due to a lessening of the stigmatization associated with cosmetic surgery combined with an increasing level of dissatisfaction with appearance. A 1985 body-image survey of 30,000 American adults found that 34 percent of men and 38 percent of women were generally dissatisfied with their looks.[1] These percentages are up from a similar survey in 1972, which found that 15 percent of men and 23 percent of women were unhappy with their appearance. In the 1985 survey, only 18 percent of the men and 7 percent of the women surveyed were very happy with their appearance.

Younger people tend to be even more unhappy. A 1989 survey of college students found that 70 percent were dissatisfied with some aspect of their body and 46 percent were preoccupied with the supposed defect.[2] Generally, as young girls get older, they become increasingly dissatisfied with their body, although girls who mature later than their peers tend to like their appearance better. *Newsweek* reported findings from a study by researchers at the University of Arizona (published in the journal *Human Organization*) that 90 percent of white teenagers say they are dissatisfied with their bodies, particularly their weight, whereas 70 percent of African-American teens claim to be satisfied with their bodies. Apparently African-American children are getting a more realistic and positive message about their bodies and themselves from parents and their subculture, which proclaims that "black is beautiful." White children, on the other hand, learn that "thinner is better" and that the body can be changed to conform, if only the owner of the body is willing to diet, exercise, and perhaps even get surgery.

A 1995 study of 54 adult women who admitted inordinate concern about some part of their body indicated that thighs, abdomens, and breast size or shape were the features producing the most dissatisfaction.[3] Skin blemishes, buttocks, facial features, weight, scars, aging, hair, hips, teeth, and arms were also mentioned. In the 1985 study, women were most unhappy with the lower torso—the area from just below the waist to the knees—and with their weight. Men were most dissatisfied with the mid torso and their weight.

Often there is no objective foundation for this dissatisfaction. The 1985 survey also found that 47 percent of women and 29 percent of men who were actually of normal weight felt they were overweight. Beauty is in the eye of the beholder, and the beholder that counts is the person in the mirror. What others think has little impact on a person's self-perception if that person is convinced of a personal imperfection.

Some people seem to be susceptible to seeing problems that others don't necessarily see. Professionals whose appearance is important, such as models or actors, are likely to be sensitive to perceived flaws. Likewise, persons with a high sense of aesthetic perception are susceptible to distress about perceived deficits in appearance, more so than similarly affected people with a less keen sense of aesthetics.

Cosmetic surgery patients often see themselves as uglier than an objective judge would. In one study, resesarchers administered personality and symptom measures to 20 men and 25 women before they underwent a nose reshaping operation.[4] Photographs of these patients, together with photographs of 45 non-patients, were then rated by independent judges. Ratings the patients made of their appearance were compared to ratings made by the judges. While the judges agreed that the cosmetic surgery patients had more severe nose defects than the non-patient control group, they considered the noses of the cosmetic surgery patients to be less prominent and unattractive than did the patients themselves. Clearly, how a person with a perceived imperfection views his or her defect, and how others perceive it, do not necessarily coincide.

How slight or significant a perceived defect really is has little relationship to how psychologically troubled the possessor of the deficit is or to the amount of personal distress it causes. Those with only a minimal problem may be very self-conscious and unhappy, while those with an objectively un-attractive feature may be relatively unaffected. One study found that rhi-noplasty patients, who judges agreed had fairly unattractive noses, were not necessarily more neurotic than those with mild imperfections. However, oth-ers with only minimal defects suffered significant distress—so much so that they obsessed about being "ugly." These patients, who have excessive concern about a very small defect, are viewed by surgeons as the ones most likely to suffer post-operative difficulties.

People who think they are unattractive may act as if they are, in fact, ugly. For example, those who believe their noses are ugly may exhibit a char-acteristic pattern of thinking and behaving known as the "Psychiatric Syn-drome of the Rhinoplasty Patient."[5] Such patients are typically shy, reclusive, and anxious in social situations. They think others look down on them or are critical of their appearance. They often develop characteristic hand move-ments or hold their heads in such a way that avoids letting their noses be viewed from a particular angle.

It doesn't matter whether a person actually has a defect in appearance; if she just *thinks* she does, she is likely to feel and behave in a manner con-sistent with her belief. In one study, subjects were led to believe that they possessed a visible and negatively valued physical characteristic.[6] Even though this was not true, these people believed that others with whom they interacted judged them and then treated them badly because of this perceived deficit. Clearly, people can mis-perceive the attitudes and actions of others if they think they look different from a socially defined, acceptable standard.

Not only do people think they are treated differently if they have a cosmetic defect, but they also behave differently once this defect is corrected. One study of female orthodontic surgery patients found that 23 percent said they smiled more after surgery, 11 percent changed the way they wear makeup, and 5 percent changed their hairstyle as a result of their different look.[7] Before orthodontic correction, patients smiled less and generally tried to camouflage their perceived defect. Another study of rhinoplasty patients found that after surgery 81 percent of patients reported that they acted more positively toward strangers and new acquaintances. [8] They also felt less anx-ious about their appearance after surgery and believed that others treated them more "positively." Interestingly, judges were unable to detect any sig-nificant improvement in these patients' appearance when they were shown before-and-after photographs of them.

Even though a person has an objectively severe defect, she still may not want a corrective operation. In a study of women with varying breast sizes, one-third were not content with their breast size, regarding it as too small. Even so, they did not want an operation.[9] Perception and unhappiness alone about a cosmetic defect is not enough to take a person to the surgeon's table. The *raison d'être* of cosmetic surgery is the significant psychological distress and self-consciousness a perceived defect can cause.

Self-Consciousness

Self-consciousness is an acutely focused awareness of self that leads to awkwardness or embarrassment in the presence of others. David Harris, a consulting plastic surgeon at Derriford Hospital in England, has studied the relationship of self-consciousness and cosmetic surgery.[10] According to Harris, self-consciousness about a perceived cosmetic defect is initially induced either by comparing oneself to others, or by being teased or criticized. Once this happens and self-consciousness takes hold, a person pays more and more attention to the offending body part. The person becomes extra-sensitive to the behavior of others toward this feature. When others engage in either hostile or friendly teasing, when they stare or make remarks behind the person's back, or when interpretations are made (or could be made) of the person based on this bodily feature, self-consciousness increases. Thus, a girl with large breasts may be judged as promiscuous, a person with baggy eyelids may be seen as tired, and a person with a large nose may be thought to possess a particular ethnicity.

Chris, the 17-year-old girl with large breasts mentioned at the beginning of this chapter, reported that when she walked by groups of men, usually standing in front of a bar or working at a construction site, they often made lewd and suggestive remarks. Whenever possible, she would cross the street to avoid them, and she always wore baggy clothes to cover up. Despite these and other efforts to protect herself from such unwanted attention, sometimes she was unable to avoid situations in which she felt embarrassed about her appearance. Silently she compared herself to other girls and wished she were more normal. With continued self-comparison and repeated exposure to embarrassing situations, Chris's self-concept began to slip. She felt less and less attractive and more and more unsure of herself in social situations. It was no comfort that some of her friends envied her physical endowment and wished that they had large breasts.

Psychological research shows that intense self-focus lowers self-esteem. The more people focus on themselves, the more critical they become and the more negative they feel about themselves. The more that attention is focused on the body, the more painfully obvious become the flaws. Conforming to a more "normal" appearance takes on pressing importance. With increased self-focus, self-consciousness becomes increasingly acute.

Many people cope with (defend against) painful self-consciousness by trying to hide the offending feature from the sight of others. Various strategies of camouflage may be employed, such as wearing loose fitting clothes and rounding the shoulders to hide large breasts, wearing glasses to hide "tired" eyes, turning away the "bad" side of the face from others, covering the mouth while talking or smiling, or avoiding cameras. Certain activities may be avoided, such as going to the beach or being seen in bright light. Self-consciousness makes people retreat into a shell or keep their opinions to themselves. They avoid calling attention to themselves. Sometimes they may try to pretend not to be self-conscious. Or they may make a preemptive strike and bring up their perceived defect in conversation before someone else does in an attempt to salvage some control of their experience. Unrelenting self-consciousness can lead to seeking repeated cosmetic surgeries to erase the perceived defect and reduce the psychological pain.

As self-consciousness continues, reinforced by attempts to cope and perhaps fueled by continued self-comparison or criticism by others, self-concept suffers. Self-conscious people come to doubt their physical attractiveness and social acceptability. Depending on the part of the body perceived as deficient, their masculinity or femininity may even come into question. The instinct is to hide the self and the painful feelings. Letting others, including doctors, know how they feel about themselves brings up the fear of further derision and stigmatization. New relationships represent a danger of exposure to more criticism from others. The presence of others who are attractive invites more self-comparison, anxiety, and a sense of being "less-than." As a result of these fears, the social networks of self-conscious people become increasingly constricted. A perceived defect involving an erogenous zone of the body may cause difficulties in sexual relationships. If self-consciousness about a perceived defect develops in childhood or adolescence, it can have a serious impact on the personality structure.

Attempts to feel better about oneself often fail. Reasoning with oneself that the defect isn't so bad, that others have it worse, that significant others claim it is fine with them, or that societal standards of beauty are unfair, doesn't usually work. Thoughts take the form of "It's me. It affects everything I do, and it's never going to change" and invite depression and hopelessness. A person may rehearse negative and distorted self-statements about her physical appearance. Harris argues that cognitive reasoning fails to remove self-consciousness because the need for a normal appearance is a deep-rooted biological instinct.

Evidence for this biological explanation of concern about appearance can be found in animal behavior. One such example observed by the author was that of a large white goose whose bill was seriously deformed in an accident. The other geese in the flock, which had previously accepted him as one of their own, repeatedly drove off the goose with the deformed bill when he tried to join them. He was relegated to the fringes of the flock based solely on his appearance defect.

Despite the possibility that concern about appearance may be a deep-seated, basic instinct, some new evidence suggests that people who are overly concerned about minimal defects in physical appearance can learn to feel better about themselves with appropriate therapy.[11] Generally such therapy targets negative self-statements and attempts to modify them into more positive thoughts. Sometimes therapy involves confrontation of perceptual distortions and introduction of relaxation and stress management skills.[12]

Although promising, therapy to help people become more self-accepting would not be needed if the causes of such focused self-consciousness were better understood and ameliorated. Some research now sheds light on the origins of becoming overly concerned about a minimal defect in oneself.

The Origins of Imagined Ugliness

Although a range of body types—from thin to fat, short to tall—has always existed, the body type considered "ideal" changes over time. At various periods in history, either fatter or thinner ideals were embraced. During the fifteenth century, paintings of long-limbed ladies graced the vaulted ceilings of Gothic cathedrals. As recently as the 1830s to the 1850s, the time period of *Gone With the Wind*, slenderness was in vogue and young ladies were encouraged to strive for a tiny waist. Even so, these same women desired ample bosoms, shoulders, arms, and calves. Not long ago, the Western body ideal for females was Junoesque—tall, full-busted, full-figured, and mature. Dimpled flesh, today called "cellulite," was considered desirable.

The current culturally defined body ideal is a post-World War II phenomenon. During this period, the health industry, given impetus by insurance companies that defined ideal weights based on actuarial analyses, launched massive campaigns to persuade Americans to change their diet, reduce saturated fat, decrease "bad" cholesterol, lose weight, exercise more, and quit smoking in order to reduce the risk of heart disease, cancer, and other lifestyle diseases. Picking up these themes, the media continue to provide health-related information. With this newly found health consciousness, the sought after body ideal for both males and females is a taut, lean, muscled, "fit" body, although the standards for males are not as extreme as those applied to females.

Some feminist writers argue that while the mass media do have the power to shape perception and attitude, the real reason for the current unrealistic body ideal is the underlying cultural beliefs that affect both genders. "Our culture is swept up in a web of peculiar and distorted beliefs about beauty, health, virtue, eating, and appetite. We have elevated the pursuit of a lean, fat-free body into a new religion."[13]

Over decades, cultural ideals find expression in a variety of ways. In the 1960s, Twiggy, at five feet seven and 98 pounds, emerged as the top model. This gawky, bare-boned, adolescent figure became the ideal of female beauty to which normal women began to aspire. In the 1990s Kate Moss carries on this image. Each year Miss America has become thinner, lighter, and taller. Increasingly, women undergo liposuction, breast augmentation or reduction, and face-lifts to conform to cultural ideals. Men seek liposuction to reduce "love handles" and enhance their chest and calves to look more muscular, younger, and attractive.

Certainly cultural pressures to conform to a particular standard of beauty set the stage for comparison of self to a body ideal that is often unattainable for many. Cultural pressure alone is not a sufficient explanation for why some people become overly concerned about an imagined or minimal defect. The first and perhaps most important influence on feelings about the body is the family. Even if a significant defect in appearance exists, if the family is accepting and treats the child in a normal way, a physical defect will take on little emotional significance. Conversely, if any family members are overly critical of a particular feature or of the child in general, self-consciousness will be induced, leading to low self-esteem and often to interpersonal difficulties. Even a chance remark, such as "You look very nice but you have your father's nose," can trigger the onset of excessive concern about appearance. A parent, often a mother, who is especially concerned about physical beauty and applies this criterion to a child can create a fertile ground for self-critical attitudes about the body. Some children secretly envy and compare themselves to their more attractive siblings, to whom their parents may also compare them, and this can foster concerns about appearance.

Generally, an environment that is emotionally poor and restrictive during childhood and that lacks positive physical contact can result in a person viewing her body unrealistically. Difficulties in family relations, including parental conflict, divorce, or abuse, can produce enduring feelings of being unloved and insecure, which may then be translated into body-related issues. Several studies comparing cosmetic surgery patients to general surgery patients found that the cosmetic surgery patients more often reported having a childhood home environment characterized by difficulties between parent and child, criticism, and feelings of insecurity.[14] Their parents were more likely to have been separated or divorced, or frequently one parent was dominant while the other was compliant.

Current family situations also contribute to appearance concerns. One study found evidence that cosmetic surgery patients continued to experience adverse family situations even as adults.[15] More so than general surgery patients, the cosmetic surgery patients indicated having difficulties in their marital relationships, and the general atmosphere at home was not as good as that reported by general surgery patients. In many cases, the cosmetic surgery patients had been forced to break away from long-term relationships. A distressing life event, such as a spouse's affair or a breakup with a boyfriend, can precipitate acute concerns about appearance.

The dramatic physical changes of adolescence can also play a role in the development of excessive concerns about appearance. Early or excessive breast development, acne, adiposity (excessive fat), protruding ears, late physical maturing, height, and premature thinning of the hair are just some of the conditions that contribute to self-consciousness in adolescence. Wanting to look like one's peers and not look different is important at this age. When a youngster doesn't conform to peer-defined standards, he or she is exposed to teasing and possible rejection.

Culture, childhood experiences, maturational changes, and the current social situation all contribute to some degree to the development of concerns about physical appearance. How a person perceives her body is learned.

Rather than asking "How do I look?" a more relevant question is "How have I been taught to see myself?" These days some people may be learning to feel that acceptance of a physical imperfection is almost a cultural taboo.

Some contend that the American worship of beauty is antithetical to freedom and equality for women because it dictates women's behavior, not their appearance.[16] This argument overlooks the fact that appearance is social currency for both men and women, although its value is greater for women.

The Social Importance of Appearance

Looks count. Throughout history, among both humans and other animals, looks count. Birds ruffle their bright plumage to attract females. Deformed animals are driven off by their kind. Appearance plays a role in sexual attraction and affiliation. The judgment of *beauty*, however, is solely an activity of humans.[17] Beauty is not a quality that resides in the object or the person. Rather, beauty is subjective. Beauty is that quality that evokes in the observer a particular feeling.

Animals do not make determinations of beauty. Nor do they purposefully alter appearance in the pursuit of beauty. In contrast, humans in various times and places have put plates in lips, hoops in earlobes, multiple rings around the neck, and scarred the skin to achieve a culturally defined standard of beauty. In prior centuries, the feet of Chinese women were bound tightly to achieve a fashionable look (and increase the woman's chances of a good marriage). In the nineteenth century, the beautiful female body was tightly corseted, producing difficulty breathing and physical discomfort. Cosmetics and clothing continue to be employed in the pursuit of beauty.

What constitutes physical attractiveness varies from culture to culture and over time. With the rise of mass media, American and Western cultures have developed a more uniform standard for physical attractiveness than ever before. Physically fit, slim, youthful-looking "hard bodies" capture the essence of what is defined as beautiful today, at least by white Americans. This ideal is seen daily on television, in the movies, and in magazines. Increasingly, men as well as women are being held to this standard. The popular myth is that anyone can attain this ideal, if only they work out enough, eat right, and as necessary, visit the plastic surgeon. The body is now seen as malleable, changeable, correctable. Once an indulgence of the rich or famous, having a face-lift is considered *de rigueur* for the aging face. High school girls think nothing of asking parents to foot the bill for a nose job. Tummy tucks and liposuction go hand in hand with a weight reduction program.

What Is Beautiful Is Good

Research provides strong evidence for a physical attractiveness stereotype that links beauty and goodness. (A stereotype is a set of beliefs about the characteristics of members of a group. It involves a structured set of inferential relations that link a social category with personal attributes.) More than 500 scholarly articles indicate that the physical appearance of both men and women, children and adults, is evaluated with great consistency by others. Virtually everyone engages in stereotyping based on appearance. The "beautiful people" are seen as possessing a wide variety of positive personal qualities. They are assumed to be more social, outgoing, popular, likable, happy, confident, and well-adjusted. Attractive men are seen as more masculine, and attractive women as more feminine.

Three broad questions have been addressed in social psychological research on physical attractiveness: Are attractive people perceived differently than unattractive people? Are attractive people treated differently than unattractive people? Do attractive people have different characteristics (i.e., personality traits, skills, behavioral tendencies) than unattractive people? Answers to all three of these are a resounding "yes!"

The perception that "what is beautiful is good" is why beautiful people are generally treated differently or regarded as having more positive characteristics than unattractive people. Physically attractive people are seen as leading more successful and more fulfilling lives. Such perceptions are conveyed and then reinforced by cultural messages about appearance. The mass media associate beauty with good things and ugliness with bad things. In children's books and fairy tales, the wicked witch is old and ugly as well as evil, and Snow White and Cinderella are young, beautiful, and good. Advertising uses young, attractive models to enhance the image of every conceivable product. In the media, beauty is associated with valued possessions, status, power, and the good things in life.

Beautiful people generally are given preferential treatment on the basis of appearance alone. The importance of appearance is felt as early as infancy and preschool. Attractive children are preferred by parents, teachers, and peers, and are universally rated as possessing positive features of every kind. Research demonstrates that caregivers cuddle, kiss, coo, smile, and look at cute babies more than homely ones. Pretty toddlers are punished less often. Teachers pay special attention and react more positively to good-looking students. These children are more popular with their peers, get chosen first as work partners or for teams, and are more frequently picked as "best friends." Severe behavioral transgressions committed by physically attractive children are viewed as less likely to reflect an enduring disposition toward antisocial behavior.

Children who are bullied are significantly less physically attractive than those who are not bullied, and they tend to have more physical handicaps and odd mannerisms. Homelier kids, and especially those with physical deformities, are more vulnerable to being blamed, punished, and physically abused. Having certain features makes some children targets. Protruding ears can lead to teasing and ridicule. Children with a cleft lip or palate are considered by many people to be less intelligent than those not similarly afflicted. Such children play alone more often and are chased away from play groups.

They have more difficulty meeting new people and are less likely to marry as adults.

The influence of attractiveness continues into adolescence and adulthood. Although both males and females are affected by the physical attractiveness of potential dates, males tend to be more responsive to females' appearance than vice versa. For both, greater attractiveness was associated with more dating and greater satisfaction in heterosexual interactions.

Discrimination based on appearance is a fact of life in Western culture. The less physically attractive are believed to have less desirable personalities, and they frequently have less social, marital, and occupational potential. This is true for both men and women. For example in her book *Body Traps*,[18] Judith Rodin Ph.D., of Yale, cites a study conducted by business school professors Jerry Ross and Kenneth Ferris of several large accounting firms that found both salary and the likelihood of becoming a partner were more strongly related to physical attractiveness than to a graduate degree or school quality.

Beauty counts for everyone, but it counts more for women. Rita Freedman, Ph.D., in her book *Beauty Bound,* terms this phenomenon the "beauty bias."[19] Attitudes about attractiveness are applied differently to men and women. In a computer dating study in which subjects were randomly assigned to blind dates, appearance was the only characteristic that accurately predicted degree of satisfaction for both sexes. Both men and women were more pleased with their blind date if the person was perceived as attractive, but physical attractiveness of a blind date was more important to men than to women. Both sexes are judged less attractive with age, but older men are still viewed as highly masculine, whereas older women are seen as less feminine as well as less attractive. Women are more critically judged for attractiveness. They are more rewarded if they have it and more severely rejected when they lack it.

In one study, male jurors were more likely to give lenient sentences to attractive female defendants, although female jurors appeared to be less biased by good looks. Other research found that young, attractive females in mental hospitals got more private therapy. Another study found that unattractive college women go out less often than their pretty roommates, but unattractive men date just as often as handsome ones.

The "rub-off effect" refers to the status one gains by association with an attractive mate or date. Female beauty has great value, and men gain value by having an "arm charm." When an unattractive man is seen with a beautiful woman, he is judged more intelligent and successful than when seen with a plain woman. Perceptions of his character, likability, and competence are enhanced. An unattractive woman paired with a handsome man gains little social advantage. Indeed, this combination may become the object of ridicule.

Attractive women tend to marry men with higher status and higher occupational levels than their own. In the mating marketplace, women's stock in trade is physical attractiveness and men's is status, career success, power, and financial security. This is sometimes referred to as the "Jackie-Ari Phenomenon," referring to the marriage of Jacqulyn Kennedy Onasis, the beautiful former First Lady, and Aristotle Onasis, the rich but physically unappealing Greek shipping magnate. Women are aware that beauty counts heavily with men and therefore they work hard to achieve it.

Gay men are as preoccupied with their looks as women, because they face problems similar to those of women. Gay men assess dates mainly on the basis of physical appearance. Like women, gay men regard their bodies as objects of courtship and sexual attraction, more so than straight men. Gays stress physical attractiveness in their personal ads, and they complain, as do women, that they become sexually obsolete at a younger age than straight men do. (By contrast, lesbian women generally have healthier body images and are more self-accepting than gay men or straight women.)

The beauty bias was further demonstrated in a study of telephone conversations between strangers.[20] Male callers were led to think the woman they were calling was either attractive or unattractive. (In fact, there was no association between the picture shown to the caller and the actual person called.) The expectations the callers had for the woman they would be calling were assessed, and the behavior of both the callers and the called were analyzed. Men who thought the woman they were calling was attractive expected her to be more sociable, poised, humorous, and socially adept than if they expected to be speaking to an unattractive woman. More surprising, however, was the dramatic impact of such expectations on both the caller's and the responder's behavior. Independent raters of the phone calls, who did not know whether the woman being called was ostensibly attractive or unattractive, rated the behavior of the male callers of "attractive" women more humorous and encouraging, and saw these men as trying harder to get the presumably attractive woman to engage with them. In response to this treatment, the reaction of the female who was called was rated as friendlier and more responsive. If the male callers were led to think that the woman they were calling was unattractive, their demeanor on the telephone was more distant and less encouraging, and the women called responded in similar fashion. These results indicate that attractive persons are more encouraged in the development of social skills and are more likely to develop self-confidence in interpersonal relationships, because they are more likely to be encouraged and rewarded, and less likely to be rejected.

Do attractive people in fact have better personality traits, skills, or behavioral tendencies than unattractive people? Often a "self-fulfilling prophecy" or "kernel of truth" underlies the attractiveness stereotype. Because beautiful people are treated more positively, they are likely to develop higher self-esteem and see themselves as more able to achieve. This preferential treatment that attractive people receive has long-term effects. They tend to be better adjusted socially, have healthier personalities, possess a wide range of interpersonal skills that help them influence others, and feel more confident because they anticipate good treatment from others. Research finds that good looks correlate with social skills, social adjustment, and the absence of shyness and social anxiety.

Attractiveness is viewed as a source of interpersonal power and popularity, and thus a major ingredient of happiness and self-esteem. Good looks strongly imply social competence, partly because of the perception that attractive individuals are socially competent and elicit positive reactions from others. This is supported by the media's portrayal of attractiveness as critical to popularity and social attention.

Adults who are treated as attractive, valuable, and as having positive features feel more confident and capable, are more socially outgoing, and achieve greater success both socially and intellectually. Physical attractiveness has a significant impact on an individual's self-esteem. The good treatment that beautiful people receive is likely to bring out the best in them. Beauty generates positive feedback.

Having good looks is clearly an asset. By contrast, having a physical deficit, or being less than physically attractive, can lead to dire consequences. One study found that 60 percent of 11,000 criminals in America have a surgically correctable deformity compared with 20 percent of the general public. This suggests that having a physical defect may increase vulnerability to bad treatment by others and precipitate antisocial behavior in response.

The "Dark Side" of Attractiveness

There is a "dark side" to attractiveness. Attractive people are also likely to be perceived as vain, egotistical, and self-centered. People may infer that attractive individuals are exposed to more opportunities for infidelity and are less likely to be faithful. It may be assumed that good looks make it unnecessary for an attractive person to develop nurturing qualities or sensitivity to the needs of others. These concerns were aptly expressed in a song that was popular several years ago that went: "If you want to be happy for the rest of your life, never make a pretty woman your wife .... "

Generally, attractiveness in females is not linked with intellectual competence in the popular culture, and this is reflected in the stereotype of the "dumb blond." Likewise, women who become students at academically demanding universities such as Harvard and Stanford are sometimes ridiculed as ugly or less attractive. The assumption seems to be that brains and beauty are mutually exclusive.

In the workplace, physical attractiveness may invite discrimination or even sexual harassment. Although decision makers often favor hiring attractive men and women, beauty can backfire, especially for women. Good looking women doing jobs that are typically held by men or are seen as requiring masculine traits for success (e.g., competitiveness, aggressiveness) may come under scrutiny for issues unrelated to their work, or they may find themselves criticized for being unfeminine. Marcia Clark, lead prosecutor in the O. J. Simpson trial, found her clothes and hairstyle the subject of frequent analysis in the media, and her cross examination style was at times termed "complaining" or "bitchy." None of the male attorneys on either side received much attention for their dress or hairstyle, and F. Lee Bailey, while labeled "bombastic," was not called "complaining" or "bitchy." Work performance evaluations of pretty women who do masculine jobs may reflect the widespread ambivalence about changing sex roles. In addition, attractive women in the workplace may be seen to elicit more unwanted sexual advances and comments.

Limits of Good Looks

A recent investigation of the physical attractiveness stereotype found that it has limitations.[21] The stereotype is strongest when people are being judged for their sociability and popularity, especially with the opposite sex, but less so when potency, intellectual competence, integrity, and concern for others are at issue. Attractive females are significantly more successful when applying for jobs requiring lower levels of skill, but attractiveness of applicants has no effect when the job calls for intelligence and concern for others. These latter qualities are not strongly associated with good looks.

Good looks are also relatively less important when more personal information is available. Physical attractiveness is most relevant when there are no or few other cues available to evaluate another person. When there is an opportunity to get to know someone, and share experiences and feedback, physical attractiveness is a less powerful force. Looks are relatively less important in the perceptions of friends, acquaintances, family members, and co-workers, than in the perceptions of strangers. The core of the physical attractiveness stereotype is sociability and popularity. Good looks have little association with integrity, concern for others, potency, adjustment, and intellectual competence. Nevertheless, given the choice, most people would prefer to be good looking.

What Does Surgery Change?

Does cosmetic surgery change how others see the person who had the surgery, and do patients see themselves differently? Michael Kalick, Ph.D., of the University of Massachusetts conducted a pioneering study in which he showed either pre- or post-operative photographs of female cosmetic surgery patients to male raters.[22] These male judges rated the photos on a variety of dimensions. Viewing pre-operative photographs, all patients were rated as less physically attractive than average. When photographs taken after surgery were shown to judges, all post-operative patients were rated as more attractive and, with one exception, above average in attractiveness. Not only did these judges rate the post-operative photographs as more physically attractive, but those who had had cosmetic surgery were judged also to have more desirable personalities, to be better potential marital partners, and to be happier and more likeable. This "halo" effect appeared to confirm the beautiful-is-good stereotype. In addition, this study seemed to suggest that those who wanted cosmetic surgery were always objectively less than average in attractiveness before surgery, and afterward always showed improvement. Unfortunately this study had methodological problems that limited confidence in the results. The judges were male, and the pictures, which showed college-age females, were taken from plastic surgery textbooks. Such texts could be expected to publish pictures that showed dramatic differences before and after surgery.

A 1983 study by Thomas Cash, Ph.D., of Old Dominion University and Charles Horton, M.D., of the Eastern Virginia Medical School used male and female judges who viewed sets of slides of either pre- or post-operative pictures of both male and female rhinoplasty patients ranging in age from 17 to 47.[23] The judges completed questionnaires assessing six trait dimensions for each photograph. Each judge saw a mix of both pre- and post-operative images without knowing which was which. The results of the experiment supported the hypothesis that cosmetic surgery not only enhances the aesthetic appeal of most patients, but also enhances perceived personality traits.

The halo effect originally identified by Kalick was confirmed, and both male and female judges were prone to it, regardless of the age of the person in the photograph. Apparently beautiful is better, no matter what your age or who is doing the judging. Unlike Kalick's results, however, the Cash and Horton study found that 6 of 14 patients were rated below average in attractiveness and 8 above average prior to surgery. Not everyone who seeks surgery is initially unattractive. After surgery, judges saw improvement in 64 percent of the patients. Apparently cosmetic surgery does not lead to objectively visible improvement in all cases. Those who were rated as more attractive before surgery were not necessarily those with the least severe physical deficit, nor were those rated as least attractive those with the most obvious deformity. The results of the Cash and Horton study suggested that nose reshaping is not requested only by people who are clearly unattractive, nor does surgical change always leads to increased or above average appeal. Cosmetic surgery can change how favorably people are viewed by others, although this is not always the case.

Similarly, Paul Marcus, Ph.D., studied the effects of rhinoplasty on patients' perceptions of themselves, judges' perceptions of these patients, and patients' behavior toward others after nose surgery.[24] Judges did not find patients to be more attractive after surgery, suggesting that the unbiased, impersonal observer does not notice a significant improvement in appearance after surgery. However, patients believed that their appearance was improved and began behaving differently toward others. Dr. Marcus concluded that the most important change that surgery brings is an intrapsychic one. The person who thinks she looks better after surgery is less anxious in social situations and becomes more outgoing. An actual change in appearance appears to have less effect on others than on the changed behavior of the patient.

An important qualification of these results needs to be made. In all three of these studies, the raters did not know who they were rating. The judges were rating strangers. Strangers constitute a "potential" social world, whereas family, friends, and acquaintances are our actual social network. The perceptions and reactions of a person's actual social network are likely to be more important than that of a stranger. One woman was devastated when soon after her face-lift, a family friend said, "You went through all this to look like that?"

The patient's established social world of friends and significant others, rather than the potential social world of strangers, can be pivotal in deciding the patient's satisfaction with the results of surgery. (See Chapter 9 for further discussion of the social context of cosmetic surgery.) One study found that patients were unhappy with their nose reshaping when families, close friends, or casual acquaintances were critical or unsupportive of the results.[25] Negative reactions from significant others can trigger disappointment and self-blame, and feelings of vanity, guilt, anxiety, or depression. Sometimes, the negative reactions of others lead the patient to blame the surgeon or complain that a surgical error was made. In other cases, a significant other may be threatened by the increased "social marketability" of a loved one and respond in a non-supportive manner in order to restore the pre-operative level of equity in the relationship. In this case, the improvement experienced by the cosmetic surgery patient is construed as a disadvantageous shift in the power balance of the relationship.

Research suggests that cosmetic surgery usually has only a moderate impact on others' perception of the patient's appearance after surgery. Even though cosmetic surgery brings about only relatively small changes, most patients indicate they are highly satisfied with the results. Given the moderate extent of socially perceived improvement that research has demonstrated, the physical changes achieved cannot be solely responsible for the high rates of patient satisfaction that have been reported. Dramatic, socially validated improvement in outward appearance may be neither necessary nor sufficient to produce increased self-esteem, lowered self-consciousness, and reduced social inhibitions. How the patients view their results is what really counts. The real change that cosmetic surgery brings is in the patient's perception of the disliked feature.

Summary

The personal impact of a perceived defect in appearance differs from person to person. The amount of psychological pain experienced is not related to the objective severity of the deficit, but to an individual's subjective evaluation. Cosmetic surgery holds out the promise of changing one's self-assessment of the body, increasing self-confidence, and thereby improving the quality of relationships. Research shows that most people with minimal deficits often see themselves as uglier than others do.

Assessing Your Perceived Deficits

Most people are dissatisfied with some aspect of their appearance, even if they are generally satisfied with their overall appearance. The following self-test is intended to help readers assess their perceived physical assets and deficits. After completing this assessment, several questions should be answered about those bodily features regarded as deficits: How long has this feature been regarded as a deficit? What were the circumstances that caused this feature to be perceived negatively? Was this feature the source of criticism of teasing? Who made this feature the focus of criticism or teasing? What attempts are made to cover up, camouflage, or make up for this perceived deficit?

Assess Your Assets and Deficits

Instructions: Rate each of the following body features according to whether you regard it as an Asset (a feature you like or feel brings positive regard from others), a Deficit (a feature you dislike or feel brings negative regard from others), or it is Neutral (neither an asset nor a deficit).

Hair	Asset	Neutral	Deficit
Ears	Asset	Neutral	Deficit
Skin	Asset	Neutral	Deficit
Teeth	Asset	Neutral	Deficit
Eyes	Asset	Neutral	Deficit
Nose	Asset	Neutral	Deficit
Lips	Asset	Neutral	Deficit
Face as a whole	Asset	Neutral	Deficit
Neck	Asset	Neutral	Deficit
Breasts	Asset	Neutral	Deficit
Arms	Asset	Neutral	Deficit
Mid torso	Asset	Neutral	Deficit
Abdomen	Asset	Neutral	Deficit
Hips	Asset	Neutral	Deficit
Buttocks	Asset	Neutral	Deficit
Thighs	Asset	Neutral	Deficit
Knees	Asset	Neutral	Deficit
Calves	Asset	Neutral	Deficit
Weight	Asset	Neutral	Deficit
Overall appearance	Asset	Neutral	Deficit

3

In Pursuit of a
Possible Self

I remember being in my late teens or early 20s and saying that if I hadn't died by age 50, I planned to "take myself out behind the barn and shoot myself." Even at a young age, the prospect of growing old was already unappealing. When I turned 40, I began to reconsider my earlier proclamation. Aging hadn't turned out to be so bad after all. Indeed, there is some comfort from the wisdom that experience brings. In fact, aging wasn't the problem; *looking my age* was the problem. Somewhere during my 40s, I arrived at another solution and made yet another proclamation: "When I turn 50, I'll get a face-lift." Frankly, it wasn't a very considered decision. I didn't think about it deeply, or talk much to friends or family about the idea. Once proclaimed, surgery became a matter of course, an event scheduled on my calendar, along with lunches and business meetings.

Although some may give relatively little thought to undertaking cosmetic surgery, others have thought about it for a long time.

> *Paulette.* "Since I was a teenager, I've hated my nose. Every time I looked in the mirror, I'd think how out of proportion to the rest of my face it was." At 41, Paulette was a talented interior designer who had an eye for detail and proportion. Her motivation to seek

a "nose job" had endured nearly a lifetime. A few years earlier she had submitted to extensive orthodontic correction. Now she was anxious to do something about that nose.

Sometimes the desire for cosmetic surgery is stimulated by the demands of a professional career or work situation. One executive in his late 40s was advised by his superior to get a face-lift so he would better fit the corporate image. Another man, a stockbroker, felt he would be more successful if he looked "less tired." He and his wife got face-lifts together. The case of "Louise" was reported in a study of face-lift patients.

> *Louise.* In her mid 50s, Louise was an executive in a government agency. She stated that her main reason for wanting a face-lift was to look "refreshed" and a little younger. It had taken her 30 years or more to work her way up the bureaucratic ladder. "It's not like the old days," she said. "Nowadays, I not only have to compete with men, which was never all that great a problem, I have to hold my own with a lot of young, good-looking, and very, very aggressive women. Looking older and as worn-out in the morning as I feel in the evening is no help."

Another reason that some people give for wanting cosmetic surgery is based on what others think of them. One recently divorced man underwent surgery to have his penis elongated, even though its length was already within normal limits. When asked why, he said that during the breakup of his marriage, his wife told him he had never sexually satisfied her. His reason for having his penis enhanced was that if any woman ever said that to him again, he would know it couldn't be true.

Internal and External Motivation

People want cosmetic surgery for a variety of reasons. A 1969 study of 750 patients undergoing a variety of different procedures found that 59 percent wanted surgery because they felt self-consciousness about their appearance.[1] Nearly 17 percent wanted others to be more accepting of them, and another 4 percent admitted to wanting others to admire them. About 15 percent wanted to improve their professional opportunities, and 6 percent just wanted a change in appearance. In another study of 71 patients undergoing breast augmentation, surgery was seen as the solution to social or sexual problems, low self-esteem, or feeling depressed and sensitive about appearance.[2] One thousand cosmetic surgery patients in Peru were primarily motivated by wanting affection and approval from other people.[3] Adults seeking orthodontic treatment were most frequently persuaded to submit to orthodontic work because of their desire for an improved appearance.[4] Even those who said that TMJ (temporomandibular joint) problems were their primary motivation admitted that they also desired cosmetic improvement.[5] TMJ problems seemed to provide the psychological permission necessary to spend the time and money for a cosmetic change.

Motivation can be either internal or external in its origin. Those who want to improve their physical appearance to satisfy themselves are said to be internally motivated. They feel that cosmetic surgery will make them feel more attractive, self-confident, or self-accepting. Externally motivated patients want surgery to please someone else. Isaac Schweitzer, M.D., of the University of Melbourne in Australia provides a good example of an externally motivated person.[6]

> A 22-year-old single man, an arts student with a prominent jaw, requested surgery to change the shape of his jaw. He expressed no personal dislike of his jaw nor was it a source of embarrassment or self-consciousness. In fact, he was relatively satisfied with his appearance, and he was not aware of it interfering in his social relationships. Upon further questioning, it was revealed that his mother frequently expressed a dislike for the young man's jaw, which she felt looked like his father. The parents divorced as the result of the father's infidelity, and the request for cosmetic surgery to correct the jaw was the result of the mother's pressuring her son.

One study of 30 women seeking breast augmentation determined that two-thirds were motivated primarily by external reasons.[7] Often they were fearful of being scorned by sexual partners, and they avoided being nude in front of them or even female friends. Frequently they compared themselves unfavorably with others, especially sisters, although one patient compared her bust with that of her adolescent daughter. Wearing bathing suits was another source of embarrassment, as was trying on clothes. Sometimes they complained of difficulty buying clothes that fit right. In a few instances, the family physician referred the patient for surgery because of unequal breast size or other physical reasons. In addition, they were acutely aware of images in the popular media of the ideal physique. Their internal motivation derived from their personal psychological discomfort and anxiety about the appearance of their breasts. These patients frequently complained of low self-esteem, and 20 percent reported a previous history of depression. Their concerns about their physical appearance led to complaints about feeling less feminine than they wished.

In this study, 53 percent were married for the first time, 7 percent were remarried, and 30 percent were divorced at the time of requesting surgery. Of the married women, 44 percent reported being unhappily married, usually because of sexual problems in the relationship. More than half of those wanting breast augmentation reported that their dissatisfaction with their breasts began in adolescence. Slightly less than half, 43 percent, said that childbirth and/or breast-feeding led to their dissatisfaction.

Although this study identified sexual partners and external motivations as a significant source of influence, others deny this. Some women claim that their desire for breast augmentation has nothing to do with the desires of their husbands or boyfriends. Carol Lynn Mithers discussed why women want man-made breasts in a story in *McCall's* magazine. She reported the response of one such woman as "I never had any trouble getting boyfriends, and no man ever said anything negative to me about my breasts." Another said, "My husband loved my little boobs. He was perfectly happy with me the way I was." These women said that their motivation to get large breasts was entirely to please themselves and relieve their own concerns. A woman identified as Connie said, "It wasn't anything anyone else said or did, the problem was me. I'd just look at myself in the mirror and . . . ugh."[8] Nevertheless, to conclude that this motivation is entirely internally generated neglects the significant influence of American culture, which some argue "neurotically worships busts."

In fact, it is often hard to tell whether a prospective patient is primarily internally or externally motivated, except in extreme cases such as the one Dr. Schweitzer described about the man with the prominent jaw. More often, both internal and external motivations are present. Jackie's request for a breast lift and augmentation involved both internal and external sources of motivation.

> *Jackie.* "I want 'hooters.' Tony likes big hooters and mine aren't big." Jackie and Tony had been married a little over a year. It was the third marriage for each of them. Jackie said that when she turned 40, she looked in the mirror and said to herself, "My God, gravity is winning!" Everything was moving downward. Jackie was a natural beauty. She had been a Miss America contestant in the 1960s and had always taken pride in her appearance. Before 40, the most exercise she had ever engaged in was turning the dial on the TV. Her bodybuilder son suggested she take up weight lifting to counteract the gravity problem. By taking up body building, she gained ground on the aging process. Indeed, she had a figure that many 20-year-olds envied. At age 50, she was still strikingly beautiful. But no amount of weight lifting could change what breast feeding two children had done. That, and her new husband's interest in other women's breasts, led her to consider having a breast lift and augmentation.

Having cosmetic surgery to please someone else can put the patient at greater risk for developing post-operative psychological complications, and doctors are hesitant to operate on such patients. The surgeon may ask, "Who will you blame if something goes wrong?" If the answer suggests the patient is primarily externally motivated, the surgeon may advise waiting. Jackie's surgeon asked her exactly this question, and her answer was "Tony." With this realization, Jackie put off her surgery for two years until she was clear she was doing it for herself as well.

Few people are motivated only by internal or external reasons; internal and external motivations interact. Feeling better about oneself tends to make social relationships go better, and improved relationships help one feel better about oneself. The most important question is whether the motivations are realistic, that is, can the surgery reasonably be expected to provide what the patient is actually seeking?

The reasons people seek cosmetic surgery are surprisingly complex, involving both conscious and unconscious motivations. Explanations of why patients seek cosmetic surgery generally fall into one of four categories: unconscious motives, mental disorders, sociocultural influences, or consistency of self-concept.

Unconscious Motives

Plastic surgery and psychiatry first crossed paths when the Wolf Man, one of Sigmund Freud's patients, sought help because of his excessive concern about a small scar left by surgery for a cyst on his nose. Frances Cooke Macgregor, clinical associate professor of surgery at the Institute of Reconstructive Plastic Surgery, New York University, commented on the early alliance between surgery and psychiatry: "With the spread of Freudian theory and its emphasis on the unconscious, intrapsychic processes [existing or occurring in the mind or psyche] and symbolic meanings of body parts, the emotional problems of patients seeking surgery became of special interest not only to psychoanalysts and psychiatrists, but to plastic surgeons as well. For the latter, such matters as motivations, surgical addiction, castration fears, and neurotic symptoms precipitated by surgery were viewed as having particular relevance for many of their own patients who suffered psychological problems."[9]

Psychoanalytic theory and thinking provided the basis for the unconscious motives model. From this point of view, a desire to change the appearance of the body was a symptom of neurosis that pointed to an underlying, unconscious conflict, usually having to do with disturbed developmental relationships with parents. From a psychoanalytic perspective, the desire for cosmetic surgery was believed to involve the unconscious displacement of sexual or emotional conflict, or feelings of inferiority, guilt, or poor self-image, onto a body part. The chosen body part was symbolic of another body part. Thus, the nose may represent the phallus and could, as such, symbolize impotence, homophobia, castration anxiety, or similar issues.

The Wolf Man's excessive preoccupation with his nose was interpreted by Freud as symbolizing a repressed sexual conflict. Additionally, plastic surgeon John Goin and his psychiatrist wife Marcia Kraft Goin describe the symbolic significance of the nose in their textbook, *Changing the Body: Psychological Effects of Plastic Surgery:*

Consider the fact that the nose is one of the only two protruding midline anatomical structures. It undergoes a spurt of growth during adolescence. It has an orifice which sometimes emits a sticky mucous substance. Microscopically, the anatomical similarities between the nose and the penis are equally striking. Histologically, nasal mucosa resembles erectile tissue. Physiologically, both the erectile tissue of the penis and the nasal mucosa become turgid when psychic influences cause vasodilation.[10]

The Goins give many examples from history and literature that suggest that the nose is symbolically a genital equivalent for both men and women. Psychoanalysts believed that sexual conflicts are often "displaced" upward, to manifest themselves as preoccupations with the nose. A woman's desire for cosmetic surgery of the nose may reflect unconscious wishes or conflicts involving parents.[11] A request for a rhinoplasty could mean she has an unconscious and ambivalent identification with her mother and a strong identification with her father. Seeking to change her nose, symbolic of father and penis, represents the wish to strengthen her identification with the mother.

Similarly, while patients give reasons for wanting breast augmentation that indicate they want to feel more feminine, sexual, or attractive, a psychoanalytic interpretation is that the patient never fully accomplished the psychic work of identification with the mother, possibly because the mother was physically or psychologically absent or unavailable.[12] By seeking augmentation the patient is unconsciously seeking a reunion with her lost mother through narcissistic identification. Full breasts are symbols of the mother and mothering. Breasts achieved through surgical means provide the feminine self-esteem that was not acquired through adequate mothering.

A completing psychoanalytic hypothesis is that some women unconsciously experience their breast size as a measure of their father's love.[13] Psychologically, having small or inadequate breasts is experienced as punishment for having affectional and sexual feelings for their fathers. A woman's request for breast augmentation may be related to unconscious guilt for having such feelings for her father.

Similar psychoanalytic explanations are provided for other cosmetic surgery operations. Women who want a face-lift are said to be attempting to augment defenses against anxiety and depression set off by aging and a reawakening of earlier dependency conflicts.[14] A women's fear of being ugly and repulsive may be the conscious manifestation of an unconscious urge to yield to sexual temptation, providing the impetus for seeking cosmetic surgery. The development of bodily symptoms are understood to be unconsciously related to incestuous wishes or castration anxiety.

From a psychoanalytic viewpoint, symptom substitution as the result of cosmetic surgery is a concern. In 1939 other researchers investigated the effects of removing a deformity that had been used by the patient to justify his lifelong dissatisfaction and sense of failure.[15] They concluded that surgery would have little effect on underlying psychopathology. Also, fears have been expressed that surgery might remove the symptom temporarily, but a secondary neurosis or even an addiction to surgery could develop.[16]

In 1944, a two-group theory was proposed that hypothesized two kinds of neurotics—basic and situational.[17] The *basic neurotic's* motivation for cosmetic surgery is a sign of a deep, underlying psychological conflict. As such, surgery could not solve this problem and would only end in symptom substitution. Basic neurotics were believed to be at risk for developing postoperative psychological difficulties. The *situational neurotic's* personality is healthier and the neurosis is limited to the effects of the appearance flaw. Presumably, patients with a minimal defect or none were basic neurotics, and those with severe defects were situational neurotics. Subsequent research found no support for this theory.[18] Indeed, the vast majority of cosmetic surgery patients showed significant psychological improvement after surgery.

A 1950 study of 48 patients seeking cosmetic surgery of the nose claimed to find evidence of the sexual significance of the nose.[19] Their results were interpreted to mean that women were seeking "to gain or obliterate masculine attributes, while for men with homosexual conflicts, rhinoplasty accomplished symbolically a wish for castration." They concluded that requests for such surgery should be regarded as a symptom of neurosis rather than a realistic response to ugliness. Of note is the fact that despite the findings of neurosis, few unfavorable post-operative results and only one incident of psychosis were found. A number of these early studies found evidence of neurosis and personality disorder in cosmetic surgery patients. (According to the American Psychiatric Association a "personality disorder" is a longstanding pattern of perceiving, relating to, and thinking about the environment and oneself that exists across situations and causes impairment in functioning and/or subjective distress.)[20] At best 30 to 60, percent of cosmetic surgery patients were found to be "normal."

The findings of the early research and the interpretations offered of motivation for cosmetic surgery clearly reflected the bias of the psychiatric community in the mid-twentieth century.[21] Psychiatrists believed it was inherently unsatisfactory and often anti-therapeutic to attempt to solve psychological problems with biologic interventions. A request for elective cosmetic surgery was invariably seen as a symptom of psychopathology, and any psychopathology was a contraindication to surgery. Despite repeated findings of post-operative satisfaction, psychiatrists continued to make a causal interpretation between neurosis, dissatisfaction with appearance, and the desire for cosmetic surgery, *and* continued to believe that neurosis remained even after surgical alterations, thus causing problems for the surgeon. Most psychiatrists contended that cosmetic surgery was indicated if, and only if, the patient's perceived defect was objectively severe.

Criticisms have been leveled at research using the unconscious motives model, mostly because of methodology problems. Much of this research involved case studies of a single individual. When groups were studied, no control groups were included. The research used psychiatric interviews with unstated structure and varying focal points. There were poor or inadequate definitions of psychiatric symptoms and diagnoses. When questionnaires were used, they were often undefined, and nothing was reported about their validity or reliability. Methodological problems lessen confidence in the findings of this research and in the notion that the desire for cosmetic surgery can be explained by unconscious motives.

Mental Disorders

Frances Cooke Macgregor, in *Transformation and Identity*, describes a patient who was motivated for surgery by a long history of teasing and rejection because of his looks.[22] When he was first seen by a plastic surgeon, he was described as a "pain in the neck." Subsequent psychiatric evaluation yielded a diagnosis of a basic personality disturbance.

> *John.* At age 22, John had what has been called "FLK Syndrome" (funny-looking kid). His large ears stood out from the sides of his rather small head. His upper jaw protruded, making the teeth so prominent that he could not bring his lips together and, in contrast, the lower jaw receded. As a child in grammar school, his peculiar face and small, thin body provoked name-calling such as "long-legged spider," "elephant ears," and "buck teeth." In his teens, when he became interested in girls, he continued to be rejected by his peers and subjected to unmitigated humiliation. His social isolation intensified and he dropped out of school. By the time he came to the surgeon requesting correction of his ears and jaw, he was hostile, arrogant, and defensive.

The mental disorder model assumes that mental illness or psychopathology underlies the motivation for cosmetic surgery. (According to the American Psychiatric Association a "mental disorder" is a clinically significant behavioral or psychological syndrome or pattern that occurs in an individual and is associated with present distress [e.g., a painful symptom] or disability [i.e., impairment in one or more important areas of functioning] or with a significantly "increased risk" of suffering death, pain, disability, or an important loss of freedom. In addition, this syndrome or pattern must not be merely an expectable and culturally sanctioned response to a particular event, for example, the death of a loved one.)[23] Research based on this premise attempts to assess the mental status of patients who request cosmetic surgery for minimal defects and assign them a psychiatric diagnosis.

One of the first collaborative studies by a plastic surgeon and a psychiatrist using the mental disorder model was undertaken in 1934 by Undergraff and Menninger.[24] They found evidence to suggest that patients seeking "superficial" changes in appearance were very narcissistic. Freud used the term "narcissism" in several different ways, but the term is currently understood to mean a person with a personality organization characterized by inflated self-concept, an inordinate need to be loved and admired by other people, and a curious inability to show concern or empathy for others. Christopher Lasch, author of *The Culture of Narcissism*,[25] describes a narcissist as emotionally shallow, fearing intimacy, hypochondriacal, lacking in self-insight, promiscuous, dreading old age and death, and having little interest in the future.

Studies conducted in the 1960s and 1970s found high rates of personality disorders and psychological disturbances among those requesting cosmetic surgery. A 1960 study attributed an unhealthy psychiatric diagnosis to 72 percent of 98 consecutive patients requesting different types of cosmetic surgery.[26] Similarly, a study published in 1969 of 750 cosmetic surgery patients found that 62 percent had a diagnosable personality disorder and 2 percent suffered from psychosis.[27] ("Psychosis" is the inability to distinguish reality from fantasy, impaired ability to understand or evaluate the world outside the self, or even the creation of a new or distorted perception of reality. It may involve paranoid ideas, delusions, or hallucinations. Based on a distorted reality, behavior may be odd, eccentric, or outside the limits of social norms.) In fact, studies conducted in the 1960s and early 1970s tended to assign a formal psychiatric diagnosis to between 50 and 80 percent of patients studied. These psychiatric diagnoses encompassed a variety of mental disorders, and patients were frequently seen as obsessive, hysterical, impulsive, depressed, dependent, or overly independent and rigid.

Some studies didn't assign formal diagnoses, but did find evidence of personal problems. One such study of 1,500 women found that younger patients seeking a face-lift had more problems with personal adjustment and more significant family disruptions during childhood than did older patients, who nevertheless had their own problems.[28] Three age-related groups were identified.

The *emotionally dependent* group constituted 21 percent of the sample and were mainly between the ages of 29 and 39. These patients were deemed insecure and found to have difficulties meeting adult responsibilities. They tended to feel hostile toward their parents, yet dependent on them. If married, these patients were extremely dependent on their spouses. They acted more like siblings than parents to their own children. Those who were widowed, were "shattered" by their losses and unable to develop new relationships.

The *worker* group, consisting of 37 percent of the sample, was mainly between the ages of 40 and 50. These patients were very committed to their careers. Relationships with spouses were stable but distant, and the most significant relationships were with coworkers. This group demonstrated the greatest anxiety and ambivalence about growing older.

The rest, 42 percent, formed the *grief* group. Most had lost an important person in their lives within the past five years and showed signs of continuing grief. Nevertheless, this group rejected sympathy and help from others, regarding this as a sign of weakness. To some extent, this group was fearful of intimacy and dependence.

Similarly, three groups for categorizing women who seek breast augmentation were hypothesized.[29] The majority of breast augmentation patients are said to fall into the *deprived childhood* group. Women in this group have been described as having life-long doubts about their femininity and their ability to compete with other women. These doubts are attributable to an emotionally deprived childhood. According to one psychoanalytic thinker, their "depressive tendencies" are probably related to inadequate mothering and a failure to identify completely with their mother.[30]

About 20 to 30 percent of breast augmentation patients fall into the *postpartum* group. They want breast augmentation because they are unhappy with the changes that take place in breast shape after pregnancy and breast feeding. Presumably this group is psychologically healthier than the larger, deprived childhood group, because they merely want to restore a body part to what it once was.

The third and smallest group of augmentation mammaplasty patients are said to be motivated by narcissistic and exhibitionistic traits. Women in this *exhibitionistic* group are overtly sexual and seductive, and want to exploit their sexual attractiveness and compete more effectively with other women. The ranks of this groups would include women who pose in the nude, topless dancers, striptease dancers, prostitutes, and the like. Although no research has been done, this group is presumed to be the least psychologically healthy of the three described.

Even though research based on a mental disorder model has frequently found evidence of high rates of psychopathology and psychological dysfunction about those seeking cosmetic surgery, the validity of these findings is doubtful. For one thing, a psychiatric diagnosis was made on the basis of a clinical interview and as such was particularly subject to interviewer bias. Evaluators were often less than objective when making the assessments. Although increasing emphasis has recently been given to developing more objective verifiable diagnostic criteria, at the time of these early studies, criteria used to arrive at a diagnosis were "fuzzy" and imprecise.

More recent studies are of special interest because, unlike earlier studies, they have included healthy control groups. One such study compared patients undergoing breast augmentation to two groups not having surgery: one group had small breasts and the other had average size breasts.[31] Subjects were asked how they felt about their breasts and their appearance in general, and all were given personality tests. Cosmetic surgery patients were found to have more negative attitudes toward their breasts than did the non-surgery controls. Furthermore, physical appearance was more important to the cosmetic surgery patients than to the others. In contrast to the small breast control group, however, the cosmetic surgery patients' personality scores were more healthy. Presumably, dissatisfaction with appearance led the patients to seek surgery, and by taking action to eliminate their distress they may have improved their psychological profile. Nevertheless, research continued to show that cosmetic surgery patients tended to have significantly more psychopathology than non-patients, although not to the degree that earlier studies suggested.[32]

Interestingly, a comparison of studies published in the 1960s to more recent studies reveals a dramatic *decrease* in the number of patients qualifying for a psychiatric diagnosis. In fact, the percentage of patients diagnosed as normal (having no psychiatric diagnosis) in studies published in the 1970s and 1980s ranged from 57 to 86 percent. There may be several reasons for this. First, the influence of psychoanalytic thinking, which tended to focus on pathology, diminished over this time, opening the way for alternative thinking about motivation for cosmetic surgery. In addition, the use of more precise and stringent criteria for assessing psychopathology reduced the number of "false positives"—those diagnosed as having a mental disorder when they actually did not. Improved research methodology characterized by greater scientific rigor has eliminated sources of bias and error. Finally, it is conceivable that more psychologically healthy people are seeking cosmetic surgery.

Despite the fact that the majority of those seeking cosmetic surgery are "normal" psychologically, a few who seek surgery do exhibit significant psychopathology. These psychiatrically impaired cosmetic surgery patients are considered further in Chapter 5. Interestingly, even though some cosmetic surgery patients are indeed psychologically distressed before surgery, there is evidence that these same patients often show significant improvement in their symptoms after surgery![33]

Sociocultural Influences

Both the unconscious motives model and the mental disorder model emphasize the motivational influences for cosmetic surgery within the person. The sociocultural model looks outward to social pressures and cultural forces in explaining motivation for cosmetic surgery.

Culture is a body of learned patterns of behavior that a group of people have in common. It is a society's distinctive way of life. Culture is not biologically inherited; rather it is a shared tradition that is transmitted from generation to generation. In short, culture is a learned way of thinking, feeling, believing, and behaving. Attitudes toward illness, surgery, hospitalization, faith in physicians, emotional responses to pain and to treatment, in fact even certain illnesses themselves, may be entirely ethnic in origin and culture-bound.

"Sociocultural" refers to both the social and the cultural influences that contribute to a person's motivation for cosmetic surgery. The "socio" part of the term refers to concepts from both sociology and social psychology. These include the processes by which social life goes on and a child is socialized into the culture. The term encompasses individual and group differences, group dynamics, social influences, social interaction, and how these affect the individual and his behavior.

In the 1950s and 1960s, several studies investigated the social and cultural influences on motivation for cosmetic surgery. A 1967 study of reasons why patients sought nose reshaping found that more than half wanted to avoid the possibility that others might stereotype them or make negative judgments because of their nose.[34] Of 89 rhinoplasty patients, 72 percent were first- or second-generation Americans. Likewise, 65 of the 89 patients were either Jewish (59 percent), Italian (25 percent), or Armenian, Greek, Iranian, Lebanese, or Syrian (10 percent) and all had variations of what is known as an "Armenoid" nose (i.e., a nose typical of people originating from northeast Asia Minor). For all of these patients ethnocultural considerations predominated. The desire to "look American" and to avoid prejudice and discrimination played a substantial role in their motivations for surgery. The remaining 43 patients, which included Irish, German, Polish, Russian, and others, gave motivations that related to individual rather than to group identity. They complained mainly of wanting to avoid stereotyping, false perceptions of their characters, and negative reactions from others that they believed were evoked by having an unsightly or conspicuous nose.

The investigator concluded that to understand why people seek surgery "one must look beyond the explanations and interpretations found in psychoanalytic and personality theory and examine patients' problems and motivations within a larger context."[35] To overlook the role that social and cultural factors play in determining the wish for surgery misses two important points—the relationship between the patient and his social and cultural milieu, and the extent to which society brings pressure on its members to conform to its standards.[36]

Carol Leppa, with the University of Illinois College of Nursing, discusses the impact of a "body-conscious culture."[37] From Chinese foot binding practices of prior centuries to the corseted hourglass figure of recent Western society, there have always been culturally based and enforced appearance ideals, and women have been the primary focus. Although the Miss America pageant was originally conceived as a means of promoting Atlantic City, New Jersey, "Miss America" is a very visible expression of culturally defined female physical ideals, despite a recent emphasis on the contestant's talent. A narrowly defined, cultural ideal of beauty is promoted on TV, in movies, magazines, advertising, billboards, literature, and in everyday interactions with others in today's society. Aging is not viewed as a normal process but as a degenerative disease and deformity to be corrected. Rather than a normal variation of body form, fleshiness is abhorred as evidence of self-indulgence. Thus, culture forms the beliefs and attitudes that influence conformity to a cultural ideal of beauty.

In *Beauty Bound* Rita Freedman discusses the notion that beauty is sought, cultivated, and rewarded in women.[38] She argues that the motivation for cosmetic surgery must be understood as part of the woman's cultural context in which she is measured against an unfair standard. Cosmetic surgery is seen as an antidote to "appearance anxiety" and a defense against "a cultural stereotype and ... the myth of female beauty." According to Freedman, appearance anxiety is culturally based, culturally dictated, and unavoidable.

Of course, men are not free from the influences of cultural ideals. Ads for hair-loss remedies, hair transplants, and natural looking hair pieces contribute to the popularity of the cosmetic hair transplantation procedures sought by many men. Despite workouts at the gym, some men do not attain the lean, muscled look that the culture values. Pectoral implants and liposuction are the answer for some. Both men and women are beauty-bound.

Naomi Wolf, in *The Beauty Myth*, provides a political and feminist perspective about beauty and cosmetic surgery. According to Wolf, the cultural prescriptions of beauty and physical appearance, and the industries that support these (including the cosmetic surgery industry), are a means of continuing to enslave women and undermine their power by alienating them from their bodies. Despite having more money, power, opportunity, and legal recognition than ever before, women are feeling worse and worse about themselves physically. Beneath the veneer of success is "a dark vein of self-hatred," obsessions about body weight and appearance, and a terror of aging. Beauty, Wolf argues, is a political weapon invoked to impede women's advancement, and cosmetic surgery is the handmaiden that serves the goals of suppression and disempowerment of women. Wolf writes that the "beauty myth," is:

> ... not based on evolution, sex, gender, aesthetics, or God, [so] on what is it based? It claims to be about intimacy and sex and life, a celebration of women. It is actually composed of emotional distance, politics, finance, and sexual repression. The beauty myth is not about women at all. It is about men's institutions and institutional power.[39]

Wolf and those who share her concerns see cosmetic surgery, not as a means of eliminating self-consciousness and improving self-esteem, but as a money-making industry that would collapse if women stopped buying into the beauty myth. To this end she urges women to stop treating themselves as objects, to stop blaming themselves for not "measuring up," and to exhibit more compassion for themselves and other women for the strong feelings all women hold about beauty. By doing so, a gradual transformation of cultural ideals is possible.

Self-Concept

According to Robert Kegan, Ph.D., of Harvard and the Massachusetts School of Professional Psychology, self-concept is a "more or less consistent notion of a me, of the who and what that I am."[40] Self-concept is traditionally seen as a generalized view or mental representation of the self in the present that includes feelings and knowledge about one's abilities and characteristics, as well as one's physical self as a whole and as various body parts.

The self-concept is constructed creatively and selectively from past experiences, and is socially determined and constrained. It reflects personal concerns of enduring importance, and influences how new information about the self is processed. Moreover, the self-concept determines what information is noticed, what is remembered, and what inferences are drawn on the basis of this information. As a result, the self-concept organizes meaning and regulates behavior.

Self-concept begins to emerge at birth and evolves rapidly in the first two decades of life, gradually reaching a relatively stable state by adulthood. (Whether the self-concept is indeed stable or much more malleable than previously thought is the center of controversy in theories of self-concept. Some research suggests that stability is really the exception and that self-conceptions can change quite dramatically, depending on certain influences.) The building blocks of the self-concept are the child's impulses, feelings, perceptions, and experiences, modified and molded by the external influences of significant others and the world in general. When a person is criticized or devalued by important others, the self-concept suffers and self-esteem sinks.

Self-esteem is the end product of the evaluation we make of ourself and is a dynamic part of self-concept. Self-esteem increases when we perceive ourself as reaching or approaching certain goals or ideal standards, and it decreases when we perceive ourself as falling short of our ideals. When Paulette looked in the mirror, she perceived her nose as being out of proportion to the rest of her face. As a result, she didn't like her nose, and she felt self-conscious about this. She was convinced that others noticed and devalued her because of her nose. Her solution to her low self-esteem was to seek a cosmetic change. Low self-esteem is painful and usually leads to efforts to reduce the psychological discomfort.

When a particular part of the body, such as the nose or the breasts, is seen as not measuring up in some way, even though a person generally feels okay about herself, an inconsistency of self-concept results. This inconsistency produces low self-esteem, which in turn can create the motivation for cosmetic surgery. (Other alternatives include changing the self-concept to be more in line with the devalued body part, that is, degrading the self-concept, or reinterpreting the body part so it is not so disliked.) Although the cosmetic surgery patient may have a generally positive self-concept, a particular part of the body may come to be seen in a less favorable light because of social influences. For example, Jackie felt good about her appearance, but because she believed that Tony valued large, pretty breasts, and because she felt her breasts did not compare well to her personal ideal, she wanted to change this part of her appearance. By doing so, her evaluation of her breasts would come into line with her overall self-evaluation, that is, there would be greater consistency in her evaluation of all body parts.

About two months after surgery when most of the healing has taken place, the patient feels better about the body part because of its changed appearance and because of positive feedback from others. To the degree that a patient feels that there has been an improvement, self-esteem rises and the self-concept is reorganized. Overall self-esteem is more consistent.

A recent study put this self-consistency theory of cosmetic surgery motivation to the test.[41] Forty adult cosmetic surgery patients were asked about their attitudes about themselves in general and about specific body parts. Results indicated that although these patients felt good about themselves overall prior to surgery, they disliked a specific body part. Each sought alteration and enhancement of the body part so that it would be consistent with overall self-concept and self-esteem. After surgery a stable improvement in overall self-esteem as well as body part self-esteem was found.

Results confirmed that motivation for surgery arises from consciously felt inconsistent esteem of self and body part and that surgery reduced this experienced inconsistency. Investigators further concluded that most cosmetic surgery patients are normal people who are working out personal inconsistencies, and are no more neurotic than the rest of the population. Studies suggest that the consistency of self-concept explanation is a viable alternative to the unconscious motives and the mental disorder models of motivation and may be more appropriate when applied to those who are seeking cosmetic surgery today.

While providing some evidence that contradicts the notion that those who seek cosmetic surgery are psychologically disturbed, this study has some shortcomings. No men were included, and past research has indicated that male cosmetic surgery patients are notoriously more psychologically disturbed than females. Nor were any psychotic, or severely neurotic, or postoperatively dissatisfied patients included. In fact, this was a study of cosmetic surgery patients who were actually a subset of all cosmetic surgery patients; it included only those who were "least disturbed" or "most normal."

Another approach to understanding motivation for self-change (though not developed specifically as an explanation for motivation for cosmetic surgery) also relies on a self-concept theory. According to Hazel Markus, Ph.D., of the University of Michigan and Paula Nurius, Ph.D., of the University of Washington, everyone has a repertoire of "possible selves."[42] Possible selves are the ideal selves that a person thinks, wishes, or fears she could become in the future. They represent specific, individually significant hopes, fears, and fantasies. Some possible selves that might be hoped for are the thin self, the beautiful self, the rich self, the loved self, or the successful self. Dreaded possible selves could be the fat self, the old self, the alone self, the incompetent self, or the unemployed self. These various possible selves are manifestations of our goals, aspirations, motives, and fears.

Although possible selves are personal and individually created, they are also distinctly social. The range of possible selves that anyone entertains is influenced by a person's particular sociocultural and historical context, by models, images, and symbols in the media, and by a person's immediate social experiences. Mae West and Marilyn Monroe were full-figured women of the 1940s and 1950s who may have suggested a possible self for many young women of the time. Today, Kate Moss and other super-models are role models of a possible self for many young women in the 1990s.

Having a mental picture of a possible self provides the impetus for action to make that possible self a reality. The concept of "possible selves" provides the essential link between self-concept and motivation for change. The concept also provides an evaluative and interpretive context for the current view of self. When Paulette looked in the mirror, she had in mind a possible self with a beautifully proportioned nose. The self in the mirror was inconsistent with this possible self, leading her to seek surgery to change her nose. Similarly, Jackie compared her breasts to the breasts of other women and to what she saw in the media. She envisioned a new self with larger and higher breasts. Her decision to proceed with breast surgery was motivated by her vision of a more buxom possible self.

The same was initially true for Anita, though her "possible self" changed over time. When she had her first breast augmentation in 1987, she was a 26-year-old account executive for a computer firm. Standing five feet five inches and weighing 120 pounds, she had a good figure overall. "I remember that I liked myself but I kept thinking how nice it would be to be a little more endowed. My 34A cup size seemed small in proportion to the rest of my figure. I also thought it would be fun to have bigger boobs and to look and feel really sexy." When she woke up after her first surgery, Anita had 34C breasts that she reported were "just gorgeous." Anita's fantasy of becoming sexually desirable was more than realized.

> The way people looked at me, and the way I looked at myself—it was incredibly sexual. The attention that it brought was just amazing to me. I guess I didn't realize it would be that way until afterwards. I would walk into a business meeting, and people would just stare at my chest. When I was out in public, cars would drive by and people would do a double-take. At first that was all fun, but as I grew older and came to accept myself more as a person, I began to struggle with the notion that I really liked the "old me." These breasts were a symbol that got a lot of attention, but they weren't really me. I felt more and more like a fraud. I think it's different when you get your nose reshaped, because it's still all your nose, but with breasts, you are adding something that isn't you. Now I feel at peace. The lies and fraud are gone. I think it's a sign of self-acceptance.

When the silicone scare hit, Anita became alarmed and took action. In 1990 she had the original silicone gel implants replaced with smaller, saline-filled implants, which she hoped would draw less attention. Finally, in 1992, she had these removed as well, so she could return to being her "old self" again, one which felt true to her.

Secret Motivations

Patients may have secret motivations for surgery that they don't share with their doctor. In a study of 50 female face-lift patients, the investigators reported that more than half of the patients revealed unrealistic or secret motivations to the researcher but not to their surgeon.[43] Some patients purposely kept their real motivations hidden, wanting not to feel foolish or to be seen as a "good" patient, but others only became aware of their additional "real" motives when they failed to be realized. This study identified three main groups of hidden motivations.

One group gave pragmatic reasons for wanting surgery—to look better, to look less tired, to get rid of sagging skin—but secretly hoped for greater involvement with younger people or to feel (rather than look) physically younger. Patients in this group were often bitter about society's youth orientation and the ever-narrowing options available to the elderly. To them, aging brought fears of abandonment by friends, family, and society in general.

The hidden motivations for another group were related to interpersonal relationships. One such motive was to reawaken a spouse's interest and to improve the relationship. One patient in this group hoped her surgery would cure her husband's impotence, which of course it did not.

The third group consisted of miscellaneous hidden motivations that did not fit in either of the other two groups. For example, one patient hoped to get a better job via improved appearance or greater self-confidence. Another was shocked to realize that her own "vanity," rather than her altruistic nature as a caregiver (which she initially believed would be more effective if she looked refreshed), was the real reason for seeking surgery.

Sometimes, those who want cosmetic surgery are not fully aware of their real motivations. It may only be after surgery, that the real reason for surgery becomes apparent. One study described cosmetic surgery patients who desired a concrete change in their appearance through surgery in preparation for a significant life change.[44] Forty-two patients requesting a variety of different cosmetic procedures were interviewed before surgery and then one to two years afterwards. Within three to six months after surgery, four of the patients studied obtained a legal separation or divorce. None of these four gave any indication prior to surgery that such a change was planned. Furthermore, no intervening psychological crisis was known to impact the family dynamics. All four patients showed a "strikingly uniform psychodynamic pattern." All had a childhood marked by social isolation, hostile relationships with younger siblings, and an early need for security. They lacked close parental ties and sought through education to maximize their potential, gain security, and prepare themselves for separation from their families of origin.

Although they had achieved significant success in their work lives and were highly valued professionally, these patients had few long-standing friendships of significance at the time of surgery. None of them expressed any feelings of inadequacy, and none had any history of psychological problems. The investigators described two of these patients:

Allen. Allen was a 35-year-old married management consultant with a Ph.D. in physics who wanted his obviously misshapen nose corrected surgically. Allen was the older of two male children, and his early life was marked by parental unavailability and lack of affection. He saw his father as an angry, unloving, aggressive person who was dominated by his wife. Allen married the first woman he dated. His wife made few demands on him and was relatively independent financially. He saw his marriage as a calculated decision, made at the right time with an acceptable person. Although their marriage continued with no evidence of overt marital discord, Allen felt that his wife "lacked the vision of the future" at a time when he had become quite successful. Two months after a very successful nose reshaping operation, with which Allen was quite pleased, he initiated a separation from his wife, eventually divorcing her. His reasoning was that she would be unable to match his new lifestyle.

Betty. At age 22, Betty, a married dental hygienist, had an augmentation mammaplasty. A year later she requested a cosmetic rhinoplasty for an objectively minimal defect of her nose. Betty was the oldest of four girls. Even though she had been raised to highly value family life, her own family of origin lacked affection, and family members communicated indirectly and covertly with one another. Betty married her grammar school sweetheart while he was in the armed services. Over the succeeding six years, she continued her education and obtained a responsible position in a large metropolitan area. Six months after a successful nose operation, she separated from her husband, complaining that he was distant and uncommunicative. She wanted the opportunity to explore interests and social contacts that her lifestyle with her husband had not permitted.

What people think or say is their reason for wanting surgery may not be the true reason. The real, less conscious motivation may become evident only after surgery. Those who have suffered strong parental domination often need to succeed on their own terms and resolve conflicts. It would seem that Allen and Betty had significant concerns with their identity that only came to consciousness and led to life changes after cosmetic surgery. Taking action by having surgery began a series of changes that may not have been entirely conscious for either Allen or Betty. The operation served to give them permission to pursue active change in other spheres of their lives, namely separation or divorce. Initiating cosmetic surgery can signal a shift from passivity and withdrawal to activity and participation. It may serve to consolidate the patient's identity and test, in a non-threatening manner, the patient's acceptance of and competence in an active role.

Marital disruption may be a possibility associated with cosmetic surgery, especially for people who have difficulty with self-expression, a marked difference in level of achievement from a spouse, and a need to resolve conflict. This is particularly true when the request for surgery is associated with recent professional, personal, or social success.

Patient Expectations

In some cases, patients hold unrealistic expectations for what surgery can do. Assessing a patient's expectations is now seen as the single most important task of the surgeon who is evaluating a person for cosmetic surgery. The surgeon must decide if the patient's expectations are realistic and see a warning sign if the patient expects surgery to radically improve his or her life. Dr. Isaac Schweitzer relates the case of one such patient:

> *Joe.* Joe was a single, 25-year-old man living with his parents. He requested nose reshaping for a larger than normal nose. He had not worked for several years and had been leading a solitary existence. Joe regarded himself as a failure with women, but blamed this on his large nose. He mentioned unrealistic business plans for which he had no finances. Joe was convinced that with surgery his improved appearance would lead to better fortune, both with work and with women. Although his appearance was vastly improved after surgery, Joe was bitterly disappointed with the result. He now blamed the surgery for his misfortune with women and with life.[45]

In another case, a woman had a face-lift to rejuvenate her relationship with her husband, who had recently retired. Although she looked younger afterwards, she did not feel younger and her relationship with her husband did not change. She had to face the reality that her marriage had been empty and unrewarding for a long time, and cosmetic surgery was not going to fix that.

The patient's perception of the surgical outcome, rather than the reality of the outcome, determines satisfaction, and perception depends on the expectations the patient holds for surgery. Generally, patients have implicit expectations about outcome in three areas. They have expectations about the extent of change that surgery will bring. If surgeons fail to "see the defect through the eyes of the patient," the surgeon's best work may still not satisfy the patient. Likewise, if the patient expects extensive or miraculous change, the surgeon must be careful not to promise more than can be delivered. A second type of expectation relates to the emotional or psychological relief expected. Most patients give their motivation for surgery as wanting to feel better about themselves. They seek a reduction of self-consciousness, relief from depression, or repair of social or sexual inhibition. Sometimes they expect an overall change in satisfaction with life. Often they are not prepared for the transient emotional and physical distress that can accompany early recovery, although patients who have been forewarned of this have a much easier time adjusting. Finally, patients expect social and interpersonal changes as a result of surgery. They want others to admire and like them, and they often hope for improved relationships with others. Frequently patients expect enhancement of their professional careers.

In addition to expectations about the results of surgery, patients have expectations about the demeanor of the surgeon and support staff, the amount of time that will be spent on the evaluation process, and the amount of time, trauma, and pain that can be expected during recovery. Some patients need more attention than can reasonably be provided by their surgeon or support staff. When a patient feels neglected, the doctor-patient relationship will suffer. (The doctor-patient relationship is discussed in more detail in Chapter 11.) Patients should not feel rushed through a consultation or made to feel that their questions or fears are not taken seriously. Surprises in the recovery process can definitely undermine the patient's confidence in the surgeon and the surgery. Patients need plenty of advance warning about the trauma and pain to be expected, especially in early recovery.

Summary

A good number of patients who want cosmetic surgery are "normal," both when assessed through clinical interview and as measured by psychological tests. The proportion of cosmetic surgery patients that are deemed normal ranges as high as 86 percent, depending on the study. Those who present with a severe psychological disorder of psychotic proportion is rare, ranging from 0 to 16 percent of patients, again depending on the study. There is no simple causal relationship between the degree of psychopathology and the motivation for cosmetic surgery.[46]

Are You a Good Candidate for Cosmetic Surgery?

If you can honestly answer "no" to each of the following questions, you are likely to be a good candidate for cosmetic surgery.

1. Do you expect that cosmetic surgery will improve your overall life situation substantially, either by rejuvenating your relationship or

marriage, by improving your love life, or by making you a great business success?

2. Are you seeking cosmetic surgery solely to please someone else?

3. Are you currently in a "life crisis"—a recent separation or bereavement, a marriage or relationship that is dissolving, losing your job, or some unexpected personal tragedy?

4. Is the decision to have cosmetic surgery a spur-of-the-moment idea— one that you have given relatively little thought to?

5. Are you convinced there is virtually no pain or physical trauma associated with the cosmetic surgery procedure you are seeking?

6. Do you need a lot of comfort and tender loving care from a doctor or special attention from the doctor's staff?

7. If you are in therapy, have you avoided discussing the proposed surgery with your therapist?

8. If you have been in therapy, have you felt misunderstood or disappointed by most therapists?

4

"Cosmetic" Is Still Major Surgery

"I'm getting my eyes done the week between Christmas and New Year's because that's the only time I can get off work, but I'm still going to the New Year's party." Helen seemed unaware that a "simple" operation to improve the appearance of her saggy eyelids, a blepharoplasty, was indeed serious surgery.

The dictionary defines the adjective "cosmetic" as "beautifying or designed to beautify" and "for improving the appearance by the removal or correction of blemishes or deformities." Yet, the implication of the word is that whatever is "cosmetic" is superficial, trivial, or frivolous. Few people realize that cosmetic surgery is not at all superficial—it is major surgery. Although it can often be done under a local anesthetic, many procedures require general anesthesia, which has its own set of risks. Cosmetic surgery is most assuredly major surgery, even though the defect it addresses may, by objective standards, be quite minimal.

Cosmetic and Reconstructive Surgery

Cosmetic surgery (also known as aesthetic surgery) is a subset of plastic surgery. Its complement is reconstructive surgery, and together, both are known as plastic surgery. In 1992, the number of reconstructive procedures outnumbered that of cosmetic procedures by three to one.

Plastic surgery is a broad surgical specialty that is not limited to an organ system or systems, as is neurosurgery or urology. It is concerned largely, though not entirely, with the surface of the body. Plastic surgeons operate on bones, tendons, nerves, muscle, and blood vessels, as well as skin. The area of competence for the plastic surgeon extends from the top of the scalp to the soles of the feet. Plastic surgery includes both cosmetic and reconstructive surgery. The term "plastic" refers to deformities caused by disease, accident, and malformation or to surgical interventions for both aesthetic and functional reasons. The word plastic comes from the Greek term *plastikos*, which means shapeable or moldable, and thus plastic surgeons shape and mold tissue to change appearance and function.

As a subset of plastic surgery, cosmetic surgery corrects defects which the average observer would consider to be within the range of normal. It involves making the normal more normal or "better" than normal. The purpose of cosmetic surgery is to treat the psychological distress that is caused by self-consciousness.

In contrast to cosmetic surgery, reconstructive surgery attempts to bring the abnormal closer to normal. As such, it is sometimes termed "functional," because it attempts to restore function or use to a particular area of the body that has been deformed by either birth defect or injury. It is that branch of plastic surgery which is devoted to the normalization of abnormal appearance or function.

Some surgery is considered reconstructive, even though its purposes are cosmetic, for example, revision of a scar from an accident or reconstruction of a breast removed because of cancer. In many cases, there is an overlap between cosmetic and reconstructive surgery, as in the case of breast reduction. Some women who have unusually large breasts not only dislike their appearance, but can suffer physical symptoms such as constant back pain, skin breakdown in the fold under the breast, and notching from bra straps digging into the shoulder. Plastic surgery can be done for both cosmetic and functional reasons.

The house of delegates of the American Medical Association in 1974 adopted the following definition of cosmetic surgery:

> Cosmetic surgery shall be defined as: That surgery which is done to revise or change the texture, configuration, or relationship with contiguous structures of any feature of the human body which would be considered by the average prudent observer to be within the broad range of "normal" and an acceptable variation for age and ethnic origin; and in addition, is performed for a condition which is judged by competent medical opinion to be without potential for jeopardy to physical or mental health.[1]

Three groups of abnormalities of appearance are treated by cosmetic surgery.[2] Disproportionate development of features during growth, such as large, small, or irregular breasts, is one such group. Another includes body contour concerns, including abnormal distribution of subcutaneous fat that results from pregnancy or weight reduction. Examples are droopy breasts or a lax abdomen. The third group of abnormalities results from aging, for example, loose skin or loose structures of the neck, sagging skin and muscles in the face, loose skin around the eyes, sagging eyebrows, forehead creasing, and wrinkled lips.

The primary goal of cosmetic surgery is the emotional satisfaction of the patient. It involves changing patients' perceptions of themselves in order to improve their psychological functioning. To this end, a variety of operations employing various techniques are available.

Restorative, Maintenance, and Type-Changing Operations

Cosmetic surgery operations can be restorative, maintenance, or type-changing. A restorative procedure restores the body or body part to a former state. A breast lift or reconstruction is usually seen as restorative. The traditional face-lift, when done without extensive additional procedures, is a restorative operation. It restores the aging face to its former youthfulness.

A growing trend in cosmetic surgery is for individuals in the early stages of aging to get a "mini-lift" to maintain, rather than re-create, a youthful look.[3] This is a face-lift that is less extensive and is usually for patients in their 30s and 40s. According to John Owsley, M.D., a plastic surgeon in San Francisco, younger patients bruise less and heal faster. (Some surgeons dispute this notion and feel that a healthy patient who has normal clotting functions and good metabolism will do quite well, whether they are 25 or 55.) Maintenance face-lifts don't make patients look drastically different, just "fresher."

A type-changing operation actually changes the person's appearance, rather than merely restoring a youthful look. Nose reshaping is a type-changing operation, as is breast reduction, breast enlargement, or procedures such as chin or cheek augmentation. Face-lifts that change the underlying muscle structure and that involve a number of other procedures can be type-changing.

The risk of psychological difficulties is much greater when patients end up looking different and not just more youthful. Patients who look drastically different after a procedure that significantly changes their appearance must integrate their new appearance with their previous mental images of themselves. Although an adaption usually takes place with time, sometimes it does not.

In *Changing the Body: Psychological Effects of Plastic Surgery,* John and Marcia Goin reported that one of their patients was a woman in her late 60s who had a chin implant to correct a receding chin line at the same time she had a face-lift.[4] Although the patient had not complained of dissatisfaction with her chin, she accepted the doctor's recommendation for a chin implant without a great deal of thought. Objectively, the result was outstanding. Even so, the woman seemed upset. A number of months later, she confronted the surgeon in tears. "Everybody says it looks nice, but I hate it. It isn't me." The chin implant had to be removed to restore her sense of self.

The Main Cosmetic Operations

According to statistics gathered for 1992 by the American Society of Plastic and Reconstructive Surgeons (ASPRS), the five most frequently performed plastic surgery procedures for women were eyelid surgery, liposuction, collagen injections, face-lifts, and nose reshaping. The top five for men were nose reshaping, eyelid surgery, liposuction, dermabrasion, and face-lifts. For children under the age of 18, the top five procedures were nose reshaping, ear surgery, breast reduction in males, dermabrasion, and breast augmentation. Those over the age of 65 seek mostly face-lifts, eyelid surgery, chemical peels, collagen injections, and forehead lifts.

The Principal Cosmetic Surgery Operations
Procedure—*Technical Name*

Breast augmentation—*Augmentation Mammaplasty*

Breast lift—*Mastopexy*

Breast reduction—*Reduction Mammaplasty*

Buttock-thigh lift

Cheek implants—*Malar Augmentation*

Chemical peel and Dermabrasion

Chin augmentation—*Mentoplasty*

Collagen injections

Ear surgery—*Otoplasty*

Eyelid surgery—*Blepharoplasty*

Face-lift—*Rhytidectomy, Rhytidoplasty, Meloplasty*

Forehead (eyebrow) lift, coronal brow lift

Hair transplantation

Implants (calf, pectoral)

Liposuction—*Suction lipoplasty, Suction lipectomy*

Nose reshaping—*Rhinoplasty*

Overbite/jaw correction—*Orthognathic surgery*

Penis enhancement

Tummy tuck—*Abdominoplasty*

Breast Augmentation

Performed to enlarge small breasts, augmentation mammaplasty has proven to be dramatically successful in relieving self-consciousness in small-breasted patients and in restoring a feeling of normal femininity. The operation involves creating a pocket under the breast tissue, or under the muscle, and inserting an implant, a soft, plastic envelope containing a saline solution. (In the United States, silicone gel implants are no longer used for breast augmentation, despite the lack of scientific evidence that firmly links such implants to autoimmune disease.) After the operation, which is sometimes done under local anesthesia, the patient must wear an elastic bra that is specially designed to help minimize swelling and bleeding. This bra is worn night and day for a few weeks following surgery, and strenuous activity must be avoided for about six weeks after the operation.

Such surgery involves risks, one of which is the formation of a breast capsule that can contract. This process is called *capsular contracture*, in which scar tissue grows and tightens around an implant, causing it to feel hard. Several years ago, the use of silicone implants was associated with complications after surgery. The introduction of new, low-bleed, gel filled silicone implants and their placement into submuscular rather than subglandular pockets reduced the incidence of post-operative fibrous encapsulation, but silicone implants are no longer available. Saline implants and the newer textured implants are less likely to cause capsular contracture. A disadvantage of the saline implants is that they wrinkle and may not feel as natural. In addition, they are more visible than the silicone implants were. Approximately 10 percent of patients now require further treatment for fibrous encapsulation of the implant.[5] About 1 percent of patients may need to have the implants removed.

An important consideration for women anticipating breast augmentation is the effect of the operation on the performance and interpretation of breast X-rays or mammograms. The implant obscures a portion of the breast in conventional views, and the radiologist is likely to have some difficulty seeing the entire breast and effectively ruling out any worrisome changes. In addition, such surgery may lead to a decrease or loss of feeling in the nipple and breast that may or may not return.

Other serious complications of such surgery are infection or deflation of the implant, which is likely to necessitate its removal. There may be breast asymmetry despite the best efforts of the surgeon. Women who have had breast enhancement can not breast-feed, and there is often a loss of sensation in the nipple.

Breast Lift

A breast lift raises and reshapes droopy breasts that can result from pregnancy and breast-feeding or from losing a large amount of weight. Sometimes this procedure is combined with breast enlargement. To correct the sagging, an incision is made on the underside of the breast from the nipple to the base of the breast and under it, in the shape of an upside down "T." Excess skin is removed and the nipple repositioned higher on the breast. Noticeable scarring is inevitable, though the severity varies from patient to patient. Usually it can be concealed with clothing. The patient should avoid gaining weight in order to preserve the improved appearance of the breast. Nevertheless, as the body continues to age, there is a tendency for some sagging to recur.

Breast Reduction

Breast reduction reduces and recontours disproportionately large, sagging breasts (macromastia), improves appearance and often relieves chronic neck and back pain, posture problems, and shoulder grooving that commonly accompany large breasts. (Because of these problems, a portion of a breast reduction operation may be covered by insurance.) Those who undergo breast reduction may also benefit by an improvement in their self-image, greater ease in buying properly fitting clothes, and increased ability to perform in sports. Women who have had breast reduction after years of trying to cope with extremely large breasts are among the most satisfied of all cosmetic surgery patients.

The procedure is usually performed under general anesthesia, followed by a short hospital stay. Incisions are made in the breast to remove excessive tissue and to reposition the nipples. It is associated with scarring, a reduction in sensitivity of the nipples, and possibly an inability to breast-feed. Pregnancy after a breast reduction can dramatically affect the shape of the breasts, and a woman may want to consider waiting for a breast reduction until after she has borne her children.

A small proportion of patients have post-operative complications, that can include prolonged healing, unusual scarring, excessive bleeding, infection, complete or partial nipple loss, and a condition called fat necrosis. The last involves the death of cells or a portion of tissue, causing drainage of fluid from the breasts through portions of the incision, which can last for a period of days or weeks. Generally, patients with very large breast reductions are more likely to have complications than those requiring less significant downsizing. Overall, the incidence of post-operative complications when done by experienced surgeons is 3 to 5 percent.

Finally, patients who do not have adequate reduction in size are likely to experience a significant loss of shape in their newly recontoured breasts in the months and years following surgery. Breast tissue, like the rest of the body, continues to age, and skin stretches with time. In particular the skin underneath the breast can stretch, causing the breast to "fall out" from underneath the nipple, which remains in about the same place as before. This condition is called "skying of the nipple," because relative to the rest of the breast the nipple is "up in the sky."

Because skin is the only structure that supports the weight of the breast, the significant variable is the weight of the breast itself. If a very large woman seeks breast reduction, the surgeon is left in a quandary. In order to reduce the breast enough to avoid eventual shape change and skying of the nipple, the breasts would have to be reduced to a size that is out of proportion. Trade-offs have to be made. Both patient and surgeon need to recognize and accept the possibility that some shape loss is likely over time, especially if the breasts cannot be aesthetically reduced to the size that is least likely to change shape in the future.

Male Breast Reduction

A little talked about but significant operation is breast reduction for men. This could be as extensive as a mastectomy or could be accomplished with liposuction. In 1992, it was the third most frequently performed operation for males under the age of 18. Most breast reduction operations are done in men under the age of 35.

Breast development is a great source of embarrassment for the male who develops *gynecomastia,* or excessive development of the mammary glands.[6] Approximately 75 percent of teenage boys, usually between the ages of 13 and 14, undergo some breast development. In more than 90 percent of these cases, the condition resolves on its own in about a year. Although breast development is common in pubertal males, it is frequently a cause of abnormal concern. If the situation is causing significant distress to the patient and it does not resolve naturally in a reasonable period of time, a breast reduction procedure may be warranted. In young boys under the age of 10 or 11, gynecomastia is always abnormal and should be brought to the attention of the child's doctor.

In adults, gynecomastia may develop with age. About 40 percent of adult men who are usually in their 40s or 50s develop breasts, usually as the result of changes in hormones and weight gain. In obese men, breast enlargement is most often the result of fat deposition. Excess skin can mimic gynecomastia in those who lose significant amounts of weight. Gynecomastia is also common in chronic alcoholics. Younger men who use anabolic steroids for body building are also at risk for developing excessively large breasts. Although a variety of causes for gynecomastia exist, it is commonly associated with a hormonal disturbance from the ingestion of a variety of substances, including marijuana and narcotic drugs.

Buttock-Thigh Lift

Although less frequently performed, now that liposuction techniques have been developed, a buttock-thigh lift works well when patients have an extreme accumulation of fat and skin in the thigh and buttock areas, and liposuction is not enough. In this operation a large wedge of fat and skin is removed from the area of the crease between the buttock and thigh. This procedure is relatively major and should not be undertaken lightly. It requires general anesthesia, hospitalization after surgery, possibly a blood transfusion, and significant restriction of activity. Unfortunately it leaves a long, unsightly scar that may need to be revised at a later time. Complications include scarring, bleeding, infection, fat necrosis, and abnormal fluid accumulation.

Chemical Peel and Dermabrasion

Both chemical peel and dermabrasion procedures are used to treat problems with the skin surface. The chemical peel is particularly useful for restoring a youthful look to facial skin with multiple fine facial wrinkles that are not correctable by a face-lift operation. The procedure removes the outer layer of skin through the application of a caustic solution containing phenol. A superficial burn of the skin occurs. A burning sensation is experienced for several seconds after the solution is applied, followed by numbness. The area weeps and crusts over, new skin forms in the place of the previous layer, and this new skin heals in a smoother surface with the elimination of many of the fine wrinkles.

Although smaller areas, such as around the lips, can be treated in the doctor's office, a phenol peel of the entire face may be done in the hospital. After the phenol solution is applied to the full face, a mask of waterproof tape is applied to prevent the solution from evaporating and to produce a deeper and more uniform peel. Shortly after the procedure is completed, the patient begins to experience a burning sensation that gradually increases in intensity. The pain continues for the next 48 hours and frequently requires narcotic medication for relief. Ice compresses applied in the first 24 hours help to reduce the pain. On the second day, the tape mask is removed while the patient is sedated and the raw area covered with an antiseptic powder. Thereafter, the patient continues the application of the powder three times a day until the wound heals. A bland ointment is used to help loosen the crust that forms over the burned skin.

The phenol peel described here is a very aggressive peel that requires the patient to have an IV and be monitored, because cardiac arrhythmias sometimes arise. In addition to crusting over of the wound, small blisters can appear on the lips shortly after the procedure is done. The newly regenerated skin that appears is thin and delicate and has a reddish-pink color. Significant scarring is a risk and the phenol peel can actually kill the pigment producing cells that are deep in the skin, leading to pigmentation changes and white blotching. All patients experience some degree of skin bleaching and pigment change in the treated skin. Patients with dark complexions or thick, oily skin may have a significant and permanent disturbance in skin pigmentation and probably will not tan as they did before the procedure. There may be a line of demarcation between treated and untreated skin. Cosmetics can be used in about two weeks to cover up the discoloration and the demarcation line.

For these reasons, the phenol peel has fallen out of favor, and most surgeons are now using the trichloroacetic acid or TCA peel. It is a much milder peel, but the theory is that "it is better to do it over than overdo it." Repeated peels can be done to achieve the same result without the risks of the phenol peel. Another advantage of the TCA peel is that people of color can have it, whereas they should never have a phenol peel.

After a peel, patients are frequently appalled by their initial appearance. During the healing period, patients frequently complain of itching, which can persist for months. Skin pores generally appear to be more prominent after a phenol peel, but not after a TCA peel. Exposure to sun must be avoided for at least six months. Although infection and facial scarring are a possibility, these complications are relatively rare with the TCA peel.

In contrast to the chemosurgery approach of a chemical peel, dermabrasion uses a mechanical method of removing the outer layer of the skin to produce a smoother, more regular surface. Dermabrasion is most useful for smoothing pitted facial scars left by acne. The skin around the pitted areas is abraded to a lower level, reducing the relative depth of the depressed areas. Unfortunately, dermabrasion does not completely eradicate the aftermath of severe acne. It can improve the smaller, more shallow scars, but deeper pits receive little benefit. Some surgeons actually remove deep pits surgically before the dermabrasion procedure to achieve a smoother look. Dermabrasion can also be helpful in treating superficial skin blemishes and the vertical lines that appear around the lips during aging.

Dermabrasion is usually performed on an outpatient basis with local anesthesia. A motor-driven abrader, similar to the handheld motorized sander used in the application of acrylic nails, is used to "sand away" the skin to the desired level. This procedure creates something like a brush burn or minor abrasion that will heal within a few weeks. As the treated area heals, it appears intensely red, resembling a sunburn. This redness resolves over a period of time. As in the chemical peel procedure, the patient is advised to stay out of the sun, and if exposure is necessary, to use a good sunscreen. Dermabrasion can sometimes cause pigmentation disturbances, particularly, increased or splotchy pigmentation that may take months or years to resolve. Though uncommon, scarring can occur if the dermabrasion is too deep.

Cheek Implants

High cheekbones are universally considered to be a hallmark of a beautiful face. For those born without high cheekbones, malar implants are the solution; a long, narrow face can be converted into a more desirable oval shape. Made from medical-grade silicone or a variety of other materials, the implants are inserted over the existing cheek bones through incisions made inside the mouth or lower eyelid, or they can be inserted during a face-lift procedure. Post-operative swelling and bruising resolves in a few weeks, but the implants may be somewhat sensitive to the touch for several months.

Chin Augmentation and Jaw Correction

Mild to moderate degrees of chin recession can be corrected by inserting a silicone chin implant through an incision in the skin just beneath the chin or through an incision inside the lower lip. More significant degrees of recession are corrected by operating directly on the bone of the lower jaw. In severe cases, orthognathic surgery may be needed to surgically correct malformations of the jaw. Such surgery is rarely performed solely for cosmetic reasons, and the goal is usually the improvement of jaw functioning as well as appearance.

Collagen Injections

Fine wrinkles and small hollows or depressions can be treated with collagen injections. Collagen is a natural ingredient in skin, bones, and body tissues, but the collagen that is injected to treat these skin problems is manufactured from cattle skin. Prospective patients are first tested to ensure that there is no sensitivity or allergic reaction. Collagen treatments are performed in the doctor's office. Using a syringe with a very small needle, the surgeon injects the collagen directly into the wrinkles or depressions. Although the collagen is mixed with a local anesthetic that is supposed to numb the skin, in fact the injections produce stinging and a fair amount of superficial pain during the procedure. Initially, the wrinkles are "over-corrected," producing a slightly swollen line where the wrinkle was. This swelling resides in a few days, and the appearance returns to normal, although a slightly lumpy feeling to the skin remains to the touch. The results are temporary, however, lasting only a few months for many people. Collagen injections must continue to maintain improvement.

Ear Surgery for Prominent Ears

In 1992, surgery for large protruding ears was the second most commonly done procedure with children under the age of 18. It is occasionally performed on adults, usually before the age of 35. Ears reach adult proportion between the ages of 4 and 6, and most otoplasties are done on children between the ages of 7 and 12. It is a relatively simple operation, with a small incision behind the ear that allows the cartilage to be molded into a more pleasing shape. Patients must wear a bulky head dressing that completely immobilizes the ears and puts some pressure on them. The dressing prevents unusual swelling and reduces the possibility of blood clot formation, which can cause damage to the ear. Pain, itching, and disruption of the bandaging that requires rebandaging is common.[7] A full four to six weeks is required before normal activities can be completely resumed. The majority of children who have such an operation experience improved self-confidence and reduced self-consciousness.

Eyelid Surgery

"Hooded" eyelids that droop over the eye and bags under the eyes from fat accumulation create a tired appearance. Increasing age and sun damage, along with recurrent bouts of eyelid swelling, result in an appearance that looks older than a patient may feel. Although eyelid surgery may be required for functional reasons, the majority of eyelid operations are done for cosmetic reasons. Excess skin and fatty tissue are removed, usually from both the upper and lower eyelids. The operation is usually done under local anesthesia on an outpatient basis. Scars are usually well hidden and fade substantially in about six months.[8] Eyelid crease asymmetry is a frequent complication of eyelid surgery. One of the most serious complications of such surgery is the pulling away of the lower lid from the eye, which can result in persistent dry eyes. In rare cases, bleeding, infection, and blindness can occur. (Only two cases of blindness have been reported, and these occurred in the 1950s.) Eyelid surgery causes quite a lot of bruising and swelling because of the thinness of eyelid tissues, although most of this resolves within a few weeks.

Face-lift

Gravity is the culprit behind the sagging cheeks, jowls, and chicken necks associated with aging. Gradually over time, the skin and underlying tissues lose elasticity. Fat accumulates in pockets under the eyes and at the jaw. The cheek skin sags forward to create a prominent fold that starts near the nose and extends down below the mouth. The forehead tissues elongate and sag, and deep furrows develop. As the brow droops, the eyebrows impinge on the eyelid space, and together with excess eyelid skin, the eyes take on a sleepy look. Frown lines from chronic squinting fan out at the corners of the eyes. Even the nose ages: the tip starts to droop and the nostrils spread. Major reconstruction is in order.

Technically, "face-lift" refers to the procedure that tightens the skin of the neck and the lower half of the face. Often, a number of other procedures are done along with a face-lift. These can include eyelid surgery, a forehead lift, a neck lift, nose reshaping, and augmentation of cheeks or chin. Vertical lines in the lips (rhitides) must be corrected either by chemical peeling, dermabrasion, or injection of collagen. (When a number of additional procedures are also done, the face-lift can be a type-changing operation.) Most people use the term face-lift to refer collectively to the group of procedures involving the face or head that are intended to restore or maintain a more youthful appearance.

Developed in Europe around the turn of the century, the standard or "classic" face-lift involves making incisions from the front of the ears around to the back of the neck and into the hair. The skin is then separated from underlying tissue, pulled back tight, and the excess skin cut off. The rest is sewn back down, leaving scars in front of the ears. This procedure produces a taut, pulled-back appearance, sometimes termed the "Lockheed look," because it appears that the unfortunate recipient is standing behind the jet engine of an airplane running at full throttle. When combined with a forehead lift, which involves making an incision at the hairline on top of the head or just behind it and pulling up the skin, the face often takes on a surprised look. Though still frequently performed, the classic face-lift is considered to be as outdated as the beehive hairdo.

Increasingly today, the classic lift is being replaced by either the SMAS-platysma face-lift or the deep plane face-lift. John Owsley, clinical professor of plastic surgery at the University of California Medical Center in San Francisco, originated the SMAS operation in 1976. It involves revamping the underlying tissues (known as the superficial musculo aponeurotic system, or SMAS for short) as well as the skin.[9] The SMAS and the underlying structures of the face work together to give the face its animation and expression. With the SMAS technique, the subcutaneous fat and the platysma muscle are lifted along with the neck skin to provide a natural-appearing result that is not excessively tight looking. For many patients, the SMAS lift significantly alters the folds that extend vertically from the base of the nose to the corner of the mouth. It is most effective for persons with moderate laxity of muscle tone and jowls. Although claims of greater duration and improvement remain controversial among some plastic surgeons, the SMAS technique is recognized by most as a significant contribution to the field.

The deep plane procedure is reserved for those with marked muscle laxity and significant creases between the nose and cheeks. Both of these "radical" face-lifts give more dramatic and longer lasting results than the classic lift, though not without a downside. They can cost more, depending on the surgeon doing it, and recovery takes longer, often six weeks or more before a patient is presentable. General discomfort can last even longer.

Face-lifts differ in men and women. Men tend to have thicker skin than women, and the results of surgery may be more subtle than dramatic. Their denser, more vascular skin, makes them more vulnerable to developing a hematoma, a swelling filled with clotted or partly clotted blood. Because men wear their hair short, the surgeon must be careful where to make the incision and how to handle the sideburns. The male face-lift patient must accept the fact that the beard will move back onto the ear as the skin is pulled back, and he may have difficulty shaving that area.

Forehead and Eyebrow Lift

With aging, the forehead and eyebrow area gradually sags, contributing to a tired, worn look. Often the forehead lift is done in conjunction with a face-lift. Although there are several ways to lift the brow area, a common procedure is to make incisions in the scalp across the top of the head or where the hairline meets the forehead. The skin is then pulled up, the excess skin removed, and the wound carefully secured. The underlying muscles can also be adjusted to reduce wrinkle lines. As with face-lift surgery, the area of the incision will not have normal feeling after surgery, and scarring, though hidden by the hair, will be noticeable to the touch. Either permanent or temporary localized baldness can occur.

One of the latest advances in forehead and eyebrow lifts is minimal incision facial surgery, or endoscopic surgery. Using special instruments such as a "scope" with a fiberoptic light source and a small video camera that shows the area being operated on, the surgeon can avoid making the long incisions from ear to ear over the scalp that is usually necessary for this procedure. Instead, three or four punctures are created, through which the scopes and instruments are introduced to allow undermining of the appropriate areas and freeing up of the attachments around the brow. Nerve bundles are protected while allowing muscle alteration. Full suspension of the muscles is achieved by inserting screws in the outer table of the scull, which holds the brow in a higher position while it is healing. The forehead is shifted up and backward without having to remove the skin. Because it is less invasive, use of this procedure minimizes hair loss, scarring, and numbness often associated with the traditional forehead lift. The endoscopic method can also be used for lifts of the cheeks and smile lines of the face, but it does not effectively correct jowls and neck skin looseness. Although initial results with this new procedure are promising, there is a down side. It can result in a longer period of swelling and may change the shape of the lower eyelid. It also costs more. Long term effectiveness still needs to be assessed.

Hair Transplantation

Hair transplants have been performed for over 30 years. The most effective way to deal with baldness is to redistribute hair on the head. The basic procedure is to take small grafts of scalp and hair from areas that are not affected by male-pattern baldness—usually the lower back of the head, the sides of the head, or above the ears—and move these to the frontal hairline. When there is not enough hair to cover the bald area, it is possible to remove sections of the scalp skin in order to advance hair-bearing scalp forward. Hair transplantation requires several operations and can be a slow process. Usually four procedures are done in a year. The procedure is done with local anesthetic. There is likely to be redness and swelling. Sometimes there is a bleeding from one or more graft areas. After about a week, the swelling and redness disappear. In the meantime, it is important not to cover the scalp. It will probably be necessary to get over some initial embarrassment about being seen during the recovery process.

An alternative transplant technique drew a lot of attention at a recent meeting of the American Academy of Cosmetic Surgery. Anthony Pignataro,

M.D., a cosmetic surgeon in Buffalo, New York, has developed "snap-on hair." According to *Investor's Business Daily,* Pignataro's technique is the hair equivalent of dental implants. Instead of anchoring artificial teeth into the jawbone, a prosthetic hairpiece is fastened to the skull.[10] A handful of little metal sockets are placed in the skull, leaving a few bumps across the head. These protrusions act like very strong "snaps" for attaching a hairpiece. The wearer can go swimming or ride a motorcycle without a helmet and not worry about the "untimely loss" of his hair.

Implants for Men

Men's attitudes about their bodies are changing. They are increasingly body and health conscious. A decade ago men were mostly concerned about a big nose or going bald. These days, the masculine ideal is well muscled but trim with firm buttocks and proportioned legs. To achieve this look, some are going to the gym, others to the plastic surgeon. Pectoral implants, known as "Arnies," help them acquire the Schwarzenegger look without the workout. Buttock implants give them firmness, and calf implants provide the illusion of well-developed legs. Silicone implants pose the same risks and issues that breast implants do for women, including capsular contracture.

Liposuction

Liposuction, a procedure that "vacuums" away unwanted fat, was first developed in France and introduced in the United States in 1982. It is now a well-accepted and relatively simple technique that can remove localized fat and leave very small, inconspicuous scars. It is used in virtually all areas of the body, from under the eyes to the kneecaps, to eliminate problems such as a double chin, cellulite, love handles, and "riding britches," fat that has accumulated on the outside of the hips and thighs. At one time liposuction was not generally recommended for elderly or obese patients, but today patients over 50 often undergo such surgery. Though not a cure for obesity, liposuction has become an adjunct procedure for a number of cosmetic surgery operations.

Although variations exist, the basic procedure is the insertion of a cannula—a hollow metal tube connected to an external suction pump—into a small incision where fatty tissue is to be removed. The cannula is repeatedly pushed forward and drawn backward through the fatty tissue, breaking it down and then sucking up the debris through the tube. Fat cells are selectively sucked out, leaving principal nerves and blood vessels intact. Fluid loss, including blood, needs to be replaced. The treated area must be compressed for at least one month by an elasticized garment. Care must be taken not to suction out too much fat, which can leave the skin with a wavy appearance.

The procedure is sometimes done under local anesthesia without hospitalization, but generally it is done under general anesthesia. Excessive bleeding and complications from anesthesia were the most common general complications reported in one study of thousands liposuction procedures.[11]

Even though lipsuction patients commonly believe that suctioned fat cannot "grow back," in fact one study found that 30 percent of patients reported the return of fat to the same site, althought the majority of these patients gained less than 15 pounds.[12] Fat most frequently returns to the tummy, reappearing in about half of all abdominal lipectomies. Those who gain weight are most likely to have fat return to the site where it was originally removed, though fact can also be deposited at other locations in the body.

Liposuction patients commonly have to cope with post-operative symptoms that can persist a month or longer. About one in five patients have pain and numbness lasting around three months, though in some instances pain has been reported to persist for up to six years. Ten percent of patients are unable to engage in their usual activities for a while, and few suffer debilitating fatigue, which usually remits in a month or two.

Personal benefits citied by patients as accruing from liposuction include having clothes fit better, liking their bodies more, and feeling freer to be seen in a bathing suit or training gear. As a result, they often begin to take better care of themselves and generally experience an improvement in their relationships. Degree of satisfaction with the procedure varies depending on the site of the liposuction, and this is discussed further in Chapter 10.

Dissatisfaction was most frequently associated with lipectomy of the buttocks. Most complaints about liposuction are that not enough fat has been removed or that the procedure has caused irregularities in the skin surface.

Nose Reshaping

Rhinoplasty is performed to reduce the overall size of the nose, reshape a tip, remove a hump, or improve a poor angle between the nose and upper lip. Most rhinoplasty or nose reshaping procedures are done by incisions inside the nose itself, so that there are no external scars. With the patient under local anesthesia, an incision is usually made inside the nostrils and the skin is lifted off the skeleton of the nose. This provides the surgeon with access to the cartilage and bone that make up the structure of the nose. The cartilage and bone are cut, trimmed, or manipulated to reshape the nose and alter its appearance.

When the size or flare of the nostrils needs to be reduced, small external incisions are necessary, but with time the resulting scars are usually inconspicuous. The tip of the nose can be thinned by removing a small portion of the cartilage on each side. Long noses are shortened by removing some of the midline cartilage called the septum. If the nose has a hump or is too wide or misshapen, the underlying bone and cartilage need to be modified. This almost always produces post-operative swelling and discoloration of the nose and eyes. Cold compresses are applied to the nose and eyes for 24 hours after the operation to minimize swelling and discoloration, and the patient is advised to sleep with the head elevated for several weeks to help reduce swelling. The swelling may cause breathing difficulties during the early recovery period.

Light gauze packing may be put inside the nose to help control bleeding, and an external tape dressing is applied. At the end of the procedure, a splint composed of tape and a plastic or plaster overlay is applied to the nose to maintain the bone and cartilage in the new shape. Nasal packing, if used, can be very uncomfortable for patients. It may be necessary to leave the packing in for three to seven days. New types of packing allow patients to breath through the nose.

When the initial bandages are removed, there is still significant swelling, and the patient may feel very disappointed with the results. The black eyes that almost always occur are usually gone in about ten days. After about two weeks, usually 90 percent of the swelling has subsided, but the remaining swelling can last six months or more. Over the next year to 18 months, the nose can continue to change in appearance as scar tissue matures. Exposure to the sun must be avoided for at least six months to prevent increased pigmentation of the nasal skin.

A possible but relatively rare complication of nose reshaping surgery with modern techniques is breathing difficulty. This may result from a tiny perforation occurring in the mucous membrane linings and the cartilage, which can lead to occasional bleeding and crusting. Another complication is the development of fullness in the area just above the nasal tip. This is frequently related to the accumulation of scar tissue, which can create a beak-like profile of the nose.

Penis Enhancement

A cosmetic surgery phenomenon that is increasingly advertised in newspapers and magazines is penile enlargement and penile lengthening. As one advertisement declares, "Dreams *do* come true." In an article in *New Woman*, Maggie Drummond suggests that as men are increasingly regarded as sex objects, their interest in cosmetic enhancement is growing.[13] Miami plastic surgeon, Riccardo Samitier, M.D., has developed a technique that removes fat from torso by liposuction and pumps it into the penis to thicken it. A different procedure is done to make the penis look longer. This procedure is currently being done in China, though it was first described as far back as A.D. 300 in the *Kamasutra*, the Indian epic about eroticism.[14] This simple technique involves cutting the two ligaments that attach the penis to the pubic bone, allowing the penis to extend out from the body by as much as two inches. Since no actual flesh is added, the operation actually creates an optical illusion that the penis is longer. The whole process takes about 90 minutes and full recovery requires about a month.

Some predict that penile enhancement will become the most popular cosmetic procedure in the United States for men in the near future. Most plastic surgeons do not see penile enhancement as a legitimate plastic surgery technique, and multiple complications can accompany such procedures. For example, the injection of fat reportedly can turn the color of the penis yellow and cause it to be lumpy. Lengthening the penis by cutting ligaments can harm the nerves that go to the penis, and, over the long term, the penis may become shorter, rather than longer. Caution is advised in seeking such procedures.

Tummy Tuck

An abdominoplasty is the removal of excess skin that may have been stretched either by pregnancies or by obesity. Even though it is commonly called a tummy "tuck," it is not a minor operation. Abdominoplasty is performed under general anesthesia and involves several days of hospitalization, as well as strict activity limitation for several weeks after surgery.

In an abdominoplasty, a long incision is made sideways across the lower abdomen just above the pubic area. Through this incision, excess fatty tissue and skin are removed, but the belly button is preserved by bringing it out through a new opening. In some cases, muscles are pulled together, snugged up, and sutured to provide better support for the abdomen. An elastic binder is worn for a time after surgery to keep bandages in place and to reduce movement. When patients first get out of bed after surgery and for seven to ten days, they need to walk in a slightly bent-over position to avoid putting too much tension on the incisions and causing too much pain. With these precautions, pain can be minimized.

This operation can be associated with significant complications, including swelling, infection, excessive bleeding, scarring, accumulation of blood fluid, skin loss, risks from the anesthesia, and death. After surgery, patients sometimes complain about decreased sensation, numbness, or a prickling feeling in the thighs or abdomen that can last several months.

Multiple Simultaneous Procedures

Some patients don't want to endure the stress of several, successive operations; they want to get it all over with quickly. In the author's case, the surgeon proposed an option of doing the eyelid surgery first and returning later for the face-lift and forehead lift operations. Working up the courage for one operation was difficult enough; my fear was that I would not return for the second. Jeanette had a similar concern:

> *Jeanette.* "I decided I was going to do it all at once. I wanted my boobs done and my nose fixed. If I was going to be miserable, why stretch it out? I told my doctor that I wanted general anesthesia because I didn't want to remember anything from the operation."

In *Health* magazine, Ann Japenga reports the case of one woman who had a forehead lift, breast lift and augmentation, tummy tuck, and fanny lift—all at once.[15] It's hard to comprehend the pressures that must drive someone to endure so much massed pain and change, all in the pursuit of beauty and youth.

Cosmetic Surgery and Ethnic Minorities

More and more members of minority groups are seeking cosmetic surgery. Such procedures can pose special challenges because of differences in skin qualities. Asians and African-Americans generally have more supple skin than Caucasians, making liposuction more successful in these groups, since the skin more readily conforms to the changed tissue shape underneath. Members of these ethnic groups often wrinkle less and show fewer signs of aging. However, these groups tend to be more prone to developing keloids, which are dark, raised scars. Because of the danger of keloids, Asians, African-Americans, and Hispanics are not good candidates for chemical peels, which "burn off" the top layers of skin. This type of treatment can also cause significant pigment changes in darker skinned patients. Nose reshaping poses a particular problem for Asians and African-Americans, whose skin tends to be thicker and heavier. When cartilage is removed, the chances are higher that the skin on the nose won't drape properly over the remaining structure. Earle Matory, Jr., an African-American plastic surgeon and coauthor of *Ethnic Considerations in Facial Aesthetic Surgery: Preventing the Unhappy Patient*, advises members of minority groups who want cosmetic surgery to select a surgeon who has training and experience with people of color.[16]

Summary

Cosmetic surgery techniques are being developed and improved all the time. Contrary to popular belief, cosmetic surgery isn't becoming simpler and less invasive. If anything, the trend is toward procedures that are deeper, more complex, and radical. This chapter gives a brief summary of the principal cosmetic surgery operations currently in use. Although the plastic surgeon is in the best position to decide what can be done, the patient needs to have a general understanding of the technique to be used, the risks involved, and in particular, the physical trauma and complications that can be expected in both the immediate recovery period and later. Prospective patients should understand that cosmetic surgery is almost always major surgery. As such, risks and benefits need to be given careful consideration, and the decision to proceed should be made with deliberation, in consultation with the plastic surgeon and possibly a mental health consultant.

5

Who Seeks Surgery
and Why

Cher, Joan Rivers, Barbara Walters, Jane Fonda, Dolly Parton, Brigitte Nielsen, La Toya Jackson, Jackie Onassis, Betty Ford, Nancy Reagan—famous women go under the knife, almost as part of their job description. In *Health* magazine, Ann Japenga reported that in Palm Springs cosmetic surgery is promoted as a routine part of a woman's beauty regimen.[1] A chemical peel is euphemistically termed a "facial rejuvenation," and cosmetic surgery is touted by local surgeons as "a restorative process that can uplift both the body and the soul." Among the Palm Springs crowd, cosmetic surgery is perceived, not as a luxury but as a necessity. In certain circles, nearly every woman has had one or more cosmetic surgery procedures. Many time their surgeries so they have healed well by the time the party season begins. Others think nothing of going to parties with stitches still showing. These women don't choose their surgeons on the basis of academic credentials or referrals from the local medical society. They find them at charity events, grand soirees hosted by the doctors themselves, or referrals from hair stylists.

Similarly, in Beverly Hills cosmetic surgery is considered a woman's rite of passage. One woman likened it to upkeep on a car: "When you buy a car, you pay for its upkeep. Why shouldn't we do the same with our bodies?"[2] Here, women don't wait until their 50s for surgery. Liposuction in their 20s, an eye tuck at 35, and the first face-lift at 42 are commonplace. One Beverly

Hills surgeon claims that 1 in 20 patients returns to his office within a year to get more flesh "sucked, tucked, or shucked."[3]

Certainly Palm Springs and Beverly Hills are not Peoria or Baton Rouge. Nevertheless, cosmetic surgery is making inroads in the Midwest and Middle America. Today, cosmetic surgery is no longer a luxury available only to the rich and famous. Nearly 70 percent of cosmetic surgery patients have household incomes of $50,000 a year or less, and 30 percent earn less than $25,000. Ordinary women constitute the vast majority of cosmetic surgery patients.

According to *Elle* magazine, Debbie Then, Ph.D. and social psychologist at Stanford University, describes a "new world" in which plastic surgery is both acceptable and unstigmatized, it is "healthy" to "do whatever it takes" to feel better about yourself, and "women are increasingly in favor of appearance enhancement."[4] Sponsored by the Collagen Corporation, Dr. Then studied 400 women who got collagen treatments, and found they didn't list aging, career advancement, or attracting a man as their main reason for plastic surgery. These women said that feeling better about themselves was their primary motivation. Dr. Then interprets such motivation as "healthy" and "inner-directed."

In contrast to Dr. Then's point of view, *Self* magazine argues that cosmetic surgery is merely the latest panacea for dealing with a poor self-image; it has taken up where anorexia left off.[5] Both the need for cosmetic surgery and anorexia are based on a drive for perfection and control. Creativity is an alternative to cosmetic surgery that is offered by Marion Woodman, a Jungian analyst. "If more women would paint, garden, dance, and keep dream journals, they would feel more authentic within their own bodies." A face in touch with the soul may be lined, but it vibrates with life. Woodman says that cosmetic surgery can't reshape the essential *being*ness of the person. A noble sentiment, this perspective stands in stark contrast to the bumper sticker that reads: "I'd rather be getting my tits done."

Today there is an acceptance of plastic surgery that would have been hard to imagine ten years ago. Between 1981 and 1991, the number of cosmetic procedures performed increased by 69 percent. The number of people seeking cosmetic surgery has increased 10 to 15 percent yearly over the past decade. The American Society of Plastic and Reconstructive Surgeons (ASPRS), which represents 97 percent of all physicians certified by the American Board of Plastic Surgery, reports that in 1992, more than 1.5 million American men and women underwent plastic surgery. Of this number, 395,000 had elective cosmetic procedures. ASPRS surgeons performed some 59,000 eyelid surgeries, 50,000 nose reshapings, 47,000 liposuction procedures, 42,000 collagen injections, 40,000 face-lifts, and 33,000 breast augmentation operations.

Men Who Seek Cosmetic Surgery

Cosmetic surgery is not limited to women. Little attention is paid to celebrities such as Kenny Rogers and Michael Douglas who get a face-lift, chin implants, or liposuction, but increasingly the ordinary man on the street is opting for surgery to improve appearance. The taboo against cosmetic enhancement for men is disappearing. The ASPRS reported that in 1992, 14 percent of all cosmetic surgery patients were men—double that of two decades ago. Often they are not flabby couch potatoes but men who tend to their appearance by working out and keeping an eye on their diet.

An article in *New Woman* magazine gives the example of Terry, who sought eyelid surgery because his baggy eyelids made him look tired.

> *Terry.* A 29-year-old man who owns his own successful computer installation business, Terry had surgery to correct the dark bags under his eyes. "I wasn't gung ho about the operation. In fact, I put it off once. It is quite frightening when you see the bruises— and it was more painful than I expected." He went on to say, "Nowadays appearance is important, and like a lot of men, I am keen on fashion and nice clothes. Yes, there is still a stigma attached to men having cosmetic surgery, but I'm careful who I tell about it."[6]

Men have a variety of reasons for wanting surgery. With the competition in the workplace, looking good can help business and bring more career opportunities. Appearance is important for anyone climbing the corporate ladder or wanting to stay on top of the heap. A jowly neck sagging over a nice shirt or a bulging mid-section poking out from a designer suit doesn't create a perception of youthful vigor. As one executive said about his motivation for a face-lift, "When I'm presiding over a board meeting, I don't want the younger board members looking at me and thinking that I look like an old lion who's had his day. I want to be seen as a young lion, ready to challenge any of them!"

Shifting male and female roles are also having an impact. As women become breadwinners in their own right and economically independent of men, they are reversing roles and looking at men as sex objects. Increasingly, men's status and self-esteem are bound up with how they look. Sexual attractiveness is of particular importance. Men have always been concerned about the size of their penis, and penis enhancement is predicted to become the most popular procedure for men.

Appearance is of particular concern among some groups, especially gay men, models, actors, and performing artists. Gay men are judged on their physical appearance almost as stringently as are women. Models, actors, and performing artists who work before the camera are understandably sensitive about their appearance and how they come across to the viewing audience.

Despite the blurring of gender roles and the greater sanction given to efforts to improve appearance for both genders, it is still more acceptable for women to be concerned about their appearance and beauty than it is for men. As a result, a man's concerns about his appearance may be more compelling and perhaps more pathological for him to decide to go ahead with cosmetic surgery. Research on men who seek rhinoplasty operations appears to support this notion.

Men Who Get "Nose Jobs"

Traditionally, men who seek nose reshaping have been suspect.[7] Often deemed "extremely narcissistic," the male rhinoplasty patient is viewed as more psychologically unstable than female patients who want their noses reshaped. Men who get "nose jobs" are responsible for the majority of physical assaults and murders of plastic surgeons.[8]

One explanation for this phenomenon is based on an hypothesized "nose-penis relationship." According to this theory, the nose is the only projecting midline structure other than the penis, and as such it has tremendous symbolic significance as a genital equivalent. In many cultures and at different times in history, the size of the nose was equated with the size of the penis, and hence virility. But beyond symbolism, some point out that the nose is in fact sexual. The nose of both males and females contains erectile tissue similar to that of the genitalia, and the nose responds to sexual excitement.

Some claim that a rhinoplasty is related to an identity crisis or a somatic conversion of a conflict. Men undergoing an identity crisis, ranging from job frustration to social problems, may attribute their problems to their nose. Single males in their late 20s or 30s may be susceptible, especially if they are confused about their masculinity and self-image.

Despite such fears, recent research suggests that only about 15 percent of men who seek rhinoplasty in fact have significant psychiatric disturbance.[9] Compared to two decades ago, men seeking cosmetic surgery today are more likely to be emotionally stable. Most men who want their nose reshaped have either a very obvious deformity, often from trauma to the nose, or a dual problem of appearance and difficulty breathing.

Children and Teens

To the dismay of at least some psychologists and medical doctors, cosmetic surgery for children and teens is becoming hardly more exotic than braces on their teeth. In 1992 ASPRS estimated that 4 percent (13,314 patients in all) of all cosmetic surgery was performed on children under 18, and 11 percent of all "nose jobs" were done on this group.[10] The top five procedures performed on children and teens were nose reshaping, ear surgery, breast reduction in males, dermabrasion, and breast augmentation.

Why would parents subject children to often painful cosmetic surgery? A child may be born with a defect, such as a hare lip, absent or misshapen ears, or a facial deformity, or may be affected by an injury, and parents want surgery to help the child look as normal as possible and avoid or minimize rejection by others. Children's complaints about their looks can be acutely distressing to parents, who sometimes see their children as a reflection of themselves. In some cases, however, parents may be well-meaning but overbearing and overly concerned about a perceived defect. If it is a minimal defect and the child is relatively unconcerned, the parents' desire for surgery may be a projection of their own wishes and fears about acceptance. If a child voices distress, words of reassurance may be enough to lift his spirits. Alternatively, parents may ignore a child's legitimate complaint, especially if the feature in question resembles a parent's or family feature. Sorting out a legitimate complaint from one without much basis is not always easy, and it is often necessary to consider the child's developmental stage and circumstances.

Appearance and Stages of Development

Children begin to become aware of appearance between the ages of 5 and 10.[11] During this time they choose to be with other children who they find attractive and tease those they consider unattractive. A child unfortunate enough to have big ears, freckles, fat lips, small stature, a physical deformity, or obesity can become the object of derision. Children who suffer significant teasing develop self-image problems and may become socially isolated and depressed. These are serious concerns, and available remedies should be considered. For some children, cosmetic surgery can do a tremendous amount of good. Nevertheless, possible advantages need to be balanced against the fact that children under the age of 12 are generally unable to understand what cosmetic surgery involves, even after it's carefully explained to them. They may not cope well with the inevitable pain, bruising, and swelling.

Between the ages of 10 and 15, children begin to make finer discriminations based on appearance. At this stage, they become increasingly aware of their appearance and the effect it has on peers as well as adults. Some who are normal in appearance are designated by their peers as either attractive or unattractive, and the objective reasons for this may not be entirely clear. For example, a child who dresses differently or whose hair is too short or to long, or a child who acts younger than his age or is very needy, may be declared "a dork" or a similar derisive label. Behavior, as well as appearance, contributes to a child's popularity or rejection.

This early teenage period is marked by rapid growth spurts and hormonal changes. The major issues are breast development, facial development, and a change in the proportion of limbs to the rest of the body. Some boys experience breast development. Although as many as 75 percent of adolescent boys are affected to some degree, male breast enlargement can be a significant source of embarrassment. When male breast development is excessive—a condition called gynecomastia—surgery is a means of correction.[12] Girls who develop breasts earlier than their peers or who develop unusually large breasts often become self-conscious (despite the value that society places on breasts) and have a less positive attitude about their body than their peers who mature later.[13] Girls frequently have asymmetric breast development, and significant asymmetry is not uncommon. Breasts can also assume an abnormal shape, such as a tubular shape. This can lead to poor self-esteem and to the avoidance of situations that may expose this problem. Mild asymmetry may improve with time. Sometimes, though, a breast is missing entirely, due to a congenital defect, and surgery to construct a complementary breast is in order. Augmentation mammaplasty for unusually small breasts or asymmetric breasts is generally not recommended until the early 20s, because continued breast development is common even after a woman has achieved her full adult stature. In the case of excessive breast development (macromastia), it may be well to visit a surgeon early for ongoing observation of changes in breast size.

During the teenage years, the face matures to adult proportions. The nose reaches its final adult size around age 13 in girls and 15 in boys. The chin does not mature until age 18 in girls and 21 in boys. Owing to the prominent position of the nose in the face, and the visual impact it has, youngsters may decide that their nose is "weird" or "abnormal," even though it is normal. It is at this point, when adolescents are most sensitive about their appearance, that concerns may be voiced about perceived defects, and teens and/or parents may begin to consider cosmetic surgery as a remedy.

The danger is that teenagers, or their parents, may have unrealistic expectations for what surgery can do. Teenagers who think that surgery will help them get back their former girlfriend or boyfriend are bound to be disappointed when the social results they crave do not come with their pinned ears or bobbed nose. Surgery won't solve deep-seated problems that require psychiatric attention.

In the teenage years, acne may become the major source of a self-image problem. Fortunately, there are medications that can help, and once the outbreak has passed—usually by the early 20s—cosmetic surgery can be considered. Other sources of teenage appearance distress may include obesity, tooth color, teeth misalignment, and excessively small or large stature. Generally surgeons take a wait-and-see attitude toward adolescents' requests for liposuction. A serious weight reduction effort is usually recommended for losing excess weight because liposuction on children risks promoting prematurely sagging skin later in life.

A child with a physical deformity must confront a growing sense of difference as awareness develops. If the family is supportive of the child with a significant deformity, the impact can be minimized. Similarly, if the family is critical of even the most insignificant appearance problem, the child can develop major self-image problems. Many who suffer from an eating disorder were teased or criticized as youngsters for their eating habits or weight. The family's opinion of a child and their concepts of "normal" will play an important role in whether a child develops a perceived deficit and whether cosmetic surgery is sought as a solution. In some cases, surgery is warranted.

Nose Reshaping

Rhinoplasty is the most frequently performed cosmetic surgery for those age 18 and under. An adolescent girl may want a "nose job," not to get a more beautiful nose but to get rid of an "ugly" one. Her primary motivation is to blend with peers and not stand out because of an unattractive feature. On the other hand, an adolescent male may want rhinoplasty to correct an injury or a nasal deformity that makes breathing difficult, rather than to correct a less than perfect nose. Nose reshaping is not recommended until the teen's nose is at least 90 percent fully grown. In some parts of the country, having nasal surgery is not unusual for teens. Although there are few studies, anecdotal evidence suggests that many teens are happy with the results of their surgery.

Ear Surgery

Prominent ear correction in children is a routine procedure in plastic surgery.[14] In 1992 it was the second most performed procedure on children under the age of 18. Of the 3,024 children obtaining ear surgery in 1992, 579 were 6 years old or younger; 1,609 were between 7 and 12; and 836 were between 13 and 18. Self-consciousness and embarrassment are the main factors that prompt such surgery. Children with prominent ears are frequently the objects of ridicule and teasing, and consequently suffer significant anxiety and distress.

Absent, abnormally shaped, or large protruding ears adversely affect the self-image of children and should be corrected relatively early in a child's development.[15] (The ear is almost adult size by age 5 or 6, and early correction is possible.) Even mildly protruding ears can cause significant distress. In a study of 30 children and adolescents, 63 percent who wanted surgery had ears that were independently rated as only moderately prominent or less.[16] Most of the children in this study wanted relief from the self-consciousness and embarrassment they felt because of their ears. Only 17 percent were unconcerned about their ears and were undergoing surgery because their parents anticipated problems if such correction did not take place.

Teasing is a common experience in childhood and adolescence. Children under the age of 13 tend to be teased the most. The more teasing a child must suffer, the more likely he is to become socially isolated. Self-consciousness can begin as early as age 4.

Surgery for the correction of prominent ears is quite successful in improving the well-being of most young patients. Nevertheless, some children do not experience relief and are dissatisfied with the outcome. These are often male children who have been markedly socially isolated prior to surgery and have high levels of distress. Children who suffer teasing before surgery are not always satisfied after surgery. Surgery does not necessarily stop teasing.

The Elderly

More and more Americans are living longer and enjoying more productive lives. In 1960 the number of people in the United States 65 years of age and older was 16.7 million. In 1985, that number jumped to 28.5 million, nearly a 71 percent increase. Since 1960, the number of people 75 years of age and older has more than doubled.

Generally "elderly" means 65 years and older. Although the elderly comprise a diverse group, they are perceived in a surprisingly singular and negative way. The stereotype of the elderly is that they are no longer a productive part of the mainstream of society. The loss of physical attractiveness that accompanies old age, along with the prevalence of crippling chronic diseases, contributes to negative attitudes and a devaluing of the elderly. Certainly the most obvious cue about age is appearance. The image of an older person with wrinkled, sagging skin, graying hair, and lax muscle tone can bring into question an otherwise functional older person's positive role in society. Looking old leads to negative labeling and treatment. Ageism takes its place alongside racism and sexism. Cosmetic surgery is a way of correcting or reversing some of this.[17]

Often there is a discrepancy between perceived age and chronological age. Many older people say they feel much younger than they look. They feel good about themselves and function well socially, but recognize that they do not look as good as they feel. Surgery provides a means of resolving the dissonance between the internal state of youngness and the visual cues of age that might be associated with negative social outcomes.

Psychologically, those who feel younger than their chronological age tend to be better adjusted and more satisfied than those who identify themselves as old. Those who perceive themselves in control of their life outcomes, based on their own efforts and abilities rather than determined by chance or the control of others, are more likely to exhibit healthy functioning.

Some elders admit to feeling old. This group of elders is no longer functioning well socially. They tend to be isolated to varying degrees, and frequently complain of feeling their age. A request for cosmetic surgery by those who feel their age or their years may be a last ditch effort to regain an internal state of well being by changing their self-perception as well as the perceptions of others. If they consider cosmetic surgery at all, they typically present numerous pre-operative anxieties about the outcome and how they will look. Because of their generalized sense of discomfort, they may find it hard to trust the surgeon. Without a positive subjective state to begin with, the hope of achieving a positive outcome is tenuous at best.

According to ASPRS, 6 percent (26,426 in all) of all cosmetic surgery procedures performed in 1992 were on people over 65. The top five most frequently done procedures were face-lifts, eyelid surgery, chemical peels, collagen injections, and forehead lifts. No breast augmentations nor any procedures to correct male-pattern baldness were recorded in 1992 for those over

65, and fewer than 20 buttock or thigh lifts were done. Apparently facial rejuvenation is paramount to elders, who have by then come to more or less accept the appearance of the rest of their body.

Ethnic Minorities

Michael Jackson and his siblings have put cosmetic surgery for minorities on the proverbial map. Although he owns up to having only two nose jobs (other sources say seven), Michael Jackson's appearance has undergone a significant metamorphosis over the past decade and a half. In a 1992 article in First magazine, David Alessi, M.D., clinical assistant professor at UCLA, offered the opinion that Michael Jackson's magical transformation is likely the result of numerous procedures, including cheek and chin implants, lip reduction and skin lightening, and probably liposuction, in addition to several nose jobs.[18] Michael's sisters La Toya and Janet have both had their noses bobbed more than once, and La Toya flaunted seemingly enhanced breasts in *Playboy* magazine. With minority celebrities seeking surgical changes and with improving prosperity, taboos against such surgery are now crumbling.

According to ASPRS, just over 20 percent of cosmetic surgery patients in 1990 were minorities—usually African-American, Asian, or Hispanic—and this market is growing, both in the United States and abroad. In Korea, nearly 80 percent of those interviewed said they hoped some day to avail themselves of cosmetic surgery. Another study of 274 Japanese found that 62 percent of those seeking cosmetic surgery were men. Unlike Caucasians, minorities of both genders are open to surgical changes of appearance. Sometimes their objective is to alter a racial characteristic. Asians may want wider eyes or eyelid folds. African-Americans may want thinner lips or smaller noses. Hispanics may want a more prominent tip to the nose and a more Caucasian contour. Mediterranean and Middle Easterners may seek a more Westernized look. More and more, however, the desire is to conform to an ethnically-defined standard of beauty.

In fact, many African-Americans seeking cosmetic surgery today tell their surgeons that they do *not* want to look like Michael Jackson. Increasingly, minorities want cosmetic surgery to improve proportions but preserve ethnic identity. Dr. W. Earle Matory, Jr., director of cosmetic surgery at the University of Massachusetts Medical Center, has been analyzing minority facial features for the elements that make them attractive.[19] It is his opinion that, while an oval-shaped face is considered ideal in Europeans, more prominent cheeks and jaws that create a rounder, fuller look are best for some other groups. African-Americans look better with wider, fuller noses. Asians should have a softer, rounder look than Caucasians. The ideal is for the altered feature to be harmonious with the rest of the face. Dr. Matory says that he personally sees very few people of color who want to change their ethnic features, and those that do are often more difficult to please. Even with a good result, they are often dissatisfied.

Minorities who seek surgery are faced with special considerations.[20] Historically, surgeons have avoided cosmetic surgery procedures in Asians and African-Americans because of the fear of inducing significant scarring or pigmentary alterations. Scarring is a particular problem. When any living tissue has been injured, whether by the surgeon's scalpel, a kitchen knife, a burn, or a dog bite, scars are formed by the growth of new cells to close the gap. Excessive repair mechanisms can be stimulated, leading to keloid and hypertrophic scarring. Whether the wound is superficial or deep the body musters an inflammatory response, bringing white blood cells and antibodies to the area to help destroy or expel intruders such as infectious organisms and dead cells. As the inflammation subsides, the cells adjacent to the injury produce collagen fibers, and scar tissue begins to form. For unknown reasons, sometimes far more new tissue grows than is needed to heal a wound. Benign, tumor-like growths of excess tissue are called keloids. These are both unsightly and uncomfortable, and can become quite large. For example, piercing an ear can produce a keloid the size of a golf ball.

In another, more common type of scarring, the hypertrophic scar overgrows the wound and becomes raised, but not to the extent the keloid does. Unlike keloids, hypertrophic scars don't extend beyond the borders of the initial trauma site. These big, angry-looking hypertrophic scars cause pain, itchiness, or irritation and sometimes interfere with body movements, especially if they occur around joints. The raised portion may subside in time, but they usually remain an ugly problem. Hypertrophic scars most often form in children, adults under 40, and dark-skinned people after deep wounds or incisions, as well as burns.

Asians and African-Americans have an enhanced response to injury of the skin. Individuals who develop keloids generally have a genetic predisposition. Keloids commonly occur on the chest, shoulders, and ear lobes following cutaneous trauma. They are rarely located on the face, palms of the hand, or soles of the feet. Keloids are difficult to treat and may require long-term therapy. They will often recur and sometimes be larger than the initial lesion. Non-essential cosmetic surgery should not be performed on keloid-formers. Keloidectomy and scar revision are commonly requested cosmetic procedures by African-Americans. Because of fear of hypertrophic scars and keloids, fewer African-American women seek breast augmentation than do Caucasian women.

During the last two decades, nose reshaping has become one of the most frequently performed cosmetic procedures for African-Americans. Instead of wanting to alter their ethnic appearance, most blacks today who seek rhinoplasty do so for the same reason as other ethnic groups—a nose that is more congruent with their facial features. African-Americans seeking nose modification often complain of flared nostrils, prominent tip, and/or a depressed and low nasal bridge. There is a myth that the "typical" African-

American nose is broad and flattened with a rounded tip. In fact, there is tremendous variation, and there is no standard technique for reshaping the African-American nose.

The noses of African-Americans and Asians differ from the noses of Caucasians in that there is little bony and cartilaginous support of thick tissue, thus making rhinoplasties challenging. Bone grafts may be necessary. Increasingly, surgeons are careful to avoid overcorrection and creation of a nose that is racially incongruent. Complications include possible scarring, asymmetry, breathing problems, infection, and hematoma formation.

More and more African-Americans are seeking lip reduction (cheiloplasty), often in combination with rhinoplasty. Done in combination, the aim is to achieve greater facial harmony and symmetry. The way the procedure is done leaves no visible scar.

Liposuction is one of the most commonly requested cosmetic procedures among African-Americans. Keloids and hypertrophic scars can form at the site of cannula insertion. Other complications include contour defects, changes in pigmentation of the treated sites, and blood clots. Any cosmetic procedure that significantly traumatizes the skin may also result in distressing and unpredictable changes in pigmentation. This is especially common following chemical peels and dermabrasion. For this reason, dark-skinned individuals are often not good candidates for such procedures.

Fortunately for African-Americans, they are less likely than Caucasians to be affected by hair loss and baldness, and therefore far fewer seek hair transplants. Initially, African-Americans were discouraged from obtaining hair transplants because of the potential for developing post-surgical keloid scars. In fact, scalp keloids are less common, and African-Americans should not be uniformly excluded from having hair transplants for this reason. It is possible to have a test graft in the recipient area in a place that can be camouflaged to check for scarring tendency. If healing is normal after three months, the operation can go ahead.

It is a myth that *all* Asian or African-American patients develop keloids or pigmentation problems after surgery. In patients with a history of keloid formation or hypertrophic scarring, elective cosmetic procedures should be either avoided or undertaken with extreme caution. Minorities without such a history and who show a good healing response can feel comfortable obtaining cosmetic surgery.

Psychiatrically Impaired Cosmetic Surgery Patients

Even though most people who seek cosmetic surgery are "normal" and do not warrant a psychiatric diagnosis, some psychologically troubled people do seek cosmetic surgery. These include people who are psychotic, delusional, paranoid, or depressed, or who have a personality disorder. In some cases, those who seek cosmetic surgery suffer from body dysmorphic disorder (BDD). Victims of child abuse and individuals who have an eating disorder are also over-represented among cosmetic surgery patients.

Psychotic or Delusional Patients

Schizophrenia includes a variety of disorders that have certain characteristic psychotic symptoms. These can include delusions about some aspect of the body (one schizophrenic woman was convinced that her left arm was dead and belonged to someone else) or involve others (a psychotic woman who shot off her jaw in a suicide attempt was convinced that the plastic surgeon who was trying to repair the damage was part of a conspiracy to torture her).

A psychotic disorder is not always a contraindication for cosmetic surgery. When the patient's delusion does not involve the body part to be altered or the operation itself, proceeding with surgery may be appropriate. Even if the delusion does involve the body or the operation, surgery for severe deformities or those that impair functioning may be advisable. The schizophrenic woman who thought the surgeon intended to torture her needed several operations to create a semblance of a mouth so that she could speak a little better, though she would never be able to eat solid food again.

The Paranoid Patient

Paranoid patients are particularly difficult. Such patients may have a paranoid personality disorder or a paranoid delusional disorder. In *paranoid personality disorder,* the person is overly suspicious, distrustful, or jealous of others, but does not suffer from delusions—perceptions or beliefs that have little or no basis in reality. The most common type of *delusional disorder* is the persecutory type, in which patients believe that they, or someone close to them, are being treated badly in some way. Another type is the delusion that another person, usually of higher status, is in love with the person. Still other types are delusions that one's sexual partner is unfaithful, that one has an illness or medical condition, or that one is special in some unusual way or has a special relationship to a deity or famous person. People with a paranoid delusional disorder often seem perfectly normal except that they have beliefs that they are being conspired against, spied upon, cheated, poisoned, maliciously maligned, or harassed, even though there is no evidence for such beliefs. Small slights are likely to be exaggerated, and these suspicious patients characteristically cannot accept a forthright explanation. They are reluctant to confide or share information and are often resentful and angry. They may even resort to violence against those they believe are trying to hurt them. Usually a person's delusional system is not grossly evident initially and clues indicating that it exists are quite subtle. These patients are quite adept at concealing the disorder and may seem perfectly normal at first blush.

Illness and surgery can precipitate an exacerbation of a patient's paranoia. Michael J. Hawes, M.D., an ophthalmologist at University of Colorado Medical Center in Denver, describes one such patient he had the bad fortune to encounter.[21]

The patient was a 29-year-old female who had had eyelid surgery done by another surgeon. She complained that her lower lids were pulled down too far and that her eyes were dry and sore, which further examination indicated appeared to be a legitimate complaint. Other than refusing to give Dr. Hawes the name of the original operating surgeon, the patient seemed intelligent and reasonable. During surgery, which was done under a local anesthetic, the patient behaved as if the procedure were an assault. Afterwards she complained bitterly about her treatment. She accused the surgeon of intentionally torturing her and of conspiring with others to harm her and deform her face. Efforts to reassure her were to no avail. Soon the surgeon began receiving nuisance phone calls from the patient—first at his office and later at his home. The patient reported him to the local medical society and to the hospital and threatened to inform the local and national media of his poor treatment. He was contacted by several attorneys to send medical records. His wife was notified anonymously that he was having an affair, and the local police were told anonymously that the surgeon was a child molester. At one point the surgeon's home telephone was disconnected and attempts were made to cut off the water and power supply to his home. Eventually evidence was uncovered to implicate the patient in these sabotage attempts.

Patients with Personality Disorders

A "personality disorder" is a long-standing pattern of thinking, feeling, and behaving that is usually counterproductive in creating and maintaining satisfactory interpersonal relationships and interferes with the bearer's ability to experience a high quality of life. A number of different personality disorders have been identified and are formally recognized by mental health experts.

The person with a paranoid personality disorder has already been mentioned. Such a person attributes to the outside world or another person the thoughts, feelings, wishes, or fears that are part of himself but are unacceptable to him. In so doing, the paranoid person is able to explain uncontrollable events that might otherwise evoke feelings of helplessness and confusion. For example, "I'm not having this pain because I elected to have surgery; the surgeon is doing this to me on purpose."

Whereas the paranoid person exhibits odd thinking, the narcissistic person is dramatic and grandiose. People with a narcissistic personality disorder appear to think more highly of themselves and their abilities than is warranted by the facts. They are preoccupied with fantasies of great success, fame, or power, and expect to start at the top without commensurate achievements or credentials. They think that rules are made for others and not for them and are surprised when others get upset with their self-centered focus. The narcissistic cosmetic surgery patient is likely to expect that surgery will help her realize her grandiose fantasies of beauty and interpersonal or occupational success. When it does not, the narcissist may become filled with rage and retaliate against the surgeon. Likewise, the narcissistic person may pay scars inordinate attention and even come to see them as "mutilation," precipitating the undertaking of legal action against the surgeon.

People with an antisocial personality disorder frequently have a history of being in trouble with the law. Often they have had problems with drugs or difficulties in business negotiations. Antisocials are impulsive, reckless, and irresponsible. They tend to be cruel and hurtful to others and to think that they have the right to take what they want. Such people are oblivious to the pain they inflict on others in the course of trying to get what they want when they want it. If even minor post-operative complications occur, the antisocial person is likely to bring a lawsuit against the surgeon.

Individuals with a borderline personality disorder are volatile. One minute they idealize another person, and the next minute they hate them. Angry outbursts are followed by tearful pleas and offerings of tokens of reconciliation, only to be followed by more angry confrontations. A person with a borderline personality disorder has a great deal of difficulty creating close emotional relationships and often experiences problems with vocational achievement.[22] The borderline's sense of self is quite tenuous, and under stress this person may experience transient psychotic decompensation. Type-changing operations pose a particular problem for borderline patients, who are likely to have difficulty bringing their body image into alignment with the results of the operation.

Patients with blatant personality disorders are often denied surgery, and they end up going from surgeon to surgeon seeking further opinions. Usually they are reluctant to see a therapist who is in a position to treat their psychological problems. Other people may not have a full-blown personality disorder but may exhibit traits suggestive of a personality problem. Such patients are more likely to find a surgeon willing to operate. However, personality patterns alone do not determine either a patient's motivations for seeking surgery or responses to it. Many factors, including the special meaning patients attribute to cosmetic surgery as well as unknowable influences from the environment, also contribute.

Depression and Cosmetic Surgery

Some people may seek cosmetic surgery as a means of coping with depression. Those people most prone to depression tend to have high personal standards of performance, highly value their independence, and have difficulty allowing themselves to be cared for. When they fall short of their own high standards, they experience guilt and self-criticism. Having their activity restricted due to illness or surgery is difficult for them to tolerate. Chapter

7 describes four groups of patients whose pre-existing depression can complicate their cosmetic surgery.

Body Dysmorphic Disordered Patients

Body dysmorphic disorder (BDD), defined as a preoccupation with some imagined defect in appearance, is a little-known disorder that may be more common than once thought.[23] Although the BDD person's concerns may sound trivial, BDD can cause severe distress and impairment and lead to social isolation, inability to function in an occupation, unnecessary cosmetic surgery, and even suicide.

Individuals with BDD feel ugly and think that their physical defects are noticeable to others, even though they are quite normal in appearance. In cases where there is a minimal problem, the BDD person's reaction to it is grossly excessive. Such patients may complain of "devious-looking" eyebrows, small genitals, a "stretched" mouth, a large or misshapen head, or any one of a variety of other supposed deformities that the patient feels is unbearably ugly. One woman who was convinced she had "facial swelling" stopped going to school to avoid being seen by others,[24] and another dangerously sped through red lights on her motorcycle so that others could not see her "excessive" facial hair.[25] A young man dated only small women, thinking that his "small" penis would not be so noticeable to women of smaller build.[26]

The case of another BDD person was reported in the *American Journal of Psychiatry*.[27] A 28-year-old single white man became preoccupied at the age of 18 with his minimally thinning hair. Despite reassurance from others that his hair loss was not noticeable, he worried about it for hours a day, becoming deeply depressed, socially withdrawn, and unable to attend classes or do his schoolwork. Although he could acknowledge the excessiveness of his preoccupation, he was unable to stop it. He saw four dermatologists, but was not comforted by their reassurance that his hair loss was minor and treatment unnecessary. The young man's preoccupation and subsequent depression persisted for ten years and continued to interfere with his social life and work until he finally sought psychiatric help at the insistence of his girlfriend, who said that his symptoms were ruining their relationship.

Freud's patient, the Wolf Man was a classic case of body dysmorphic disorder. Because of his excessive concern about the state of his nose, the Wolf Man neglected his daily life and work. "His life was centered on the little mirror in his pocket, and his fate depended on what it revealed or was about to reveal" about his nose.[28]

People with BDD overfocus on one aspect of the body, which they despise and find distasteful. Sometimes they are preoccupied with different body parts at different times or with several simultaneously. Some experts suggest that the symptoms of BDD are similar to obsessional thinking, in that there are persistent, distressing thoughts that are intrusive and difficult to ignore or suppress.[29] Mirror checking and hair combing can take on the proportions of compulsive, ritualistic behaviors. Others feel that the symptoms are more akin to overvalued ideas than to obsessions. Unlike obsessive-compulsive disorder, thoughts about the ugliness of a body part seem natural to the BDD person, who acquiesces to them without much resistance. The BDD person is convinced the body part is ugly and doesn't see this conviction as at all senseless or without basis. BDD people experience a private, inner torment, because they want to appear normal but are sure that others think they are not.

BDD may be related to fear of negative social evaluation. Sufferers may be shy and experience high anxiety in social situations and try to avoid them. They fear criticism and adverse comments about their appearance. Often they are concerned that others may be looking at, talking about, or mocking their "defect." They may try to camouflage a defect with makeup, hands, hair, a hat, or other clothing. In addition, they engage in frequent comparing of their "ugly" body part with that of others or repeatedly seek reassurance that they look normal. Often they will seek unnecessary plastic surgery or the assistance of medical specialists such as dermatologists.

An estimated 2 percent of all patients who request plastic surgery suffer from BDD.[30] They may go from surgeon to surgeon requesting one procedure or another, but are rarely satisfied with the results. After surgery, they may become even more preoccupied with the same defect and seek additional operations for it, or they may focus on a new defect. One patient had four rhinoplasties and then became preoccupied with his waist, thinning hair, and sloped shoulders. Eventually, some patients become "synthetic creations of artificial noses, breasts, ears, and hips."[31]

It is difficult to tell which cosmetic surgery applicants have BDD. One tip off may be that such patients by definition have a minimal defect but have an excessive reaction to the perceived problem. Or they may request unusual procedures, such as interface surgery, which involves alteration of the hard rather than soft tissues—bone rather than skin.

One such patient was described by Michael Pertschuk, M.D.[32] A 34-year-old housewife presented with a chief complaint that her face was too broad. She was correct in that her face was rather wide, but not to the point where it would draw attention. Her perception was otherwise. She organized her time to avoid nearly all social contacts during daylight. She ventured out from her home only after dark, when she thought her deformity would be less noticeable. She had spent years researching which plastic surgeons might be able and willing to narrow the width of her skull to correct the deformity. The patient was accepted for surgery on the basis that cosmetic improvement could be achieved with minimal risk. Following surgery, the patient perceived some improvement but continued to feel deformed. Soon she resumed her search for another surgeon who could completely correct her "malformation."

Nearly 95 percent of BDD patients have severe psychopathology, including high levels of depression and dissatisfaction with their relationships and their self-concept. Women are more apt to have a body dysmorphic disorder than men, and BDD patients are predominantly unmarried. The age of onset is from early adolescence through the 20s, with 19 being the mean age. People with BDD tend to be perfectionistic, self-critical, insecure, sensitive, shy, or reserved, with obsessive-compulsive traits. Although a definitive treatment for BDD does not yet exist, sufferers can often be helped with anti-depressant medication. Cosmetic surgery does not help. Indeed, BDD is likely the reason that some patients seek repeated surgeries.

The Insatiable Patient

An "insatiable patient" is one who keeps asking for a repetition of a cosmetic surgical correction, either because she thinks the surgeon does not do a proper job or because she continues to find imperfection. From a surgical-technical point of view, the operation is a success and no mistake was made, but the patient is still not satisfied and keeps coming back for more. Dissatisfaction with her appearance continues and is followed by further requests for cosmetic surgery. The patient discredits the work of previous surgeons, while flattering the current surgeon. She may bring the surgeon photographs and drawings showing the changes she wants, and she may say that having surgery is urgent.

Isaac Schweitzer, M.D., of the University of Melbourne in Australia, gives an example of an insatiable patient with narcissistic features.[33] A handsome 22-year-old single man, who had had four cosmetic procedures in the preceding two years, asked for further surgery. He complained that his chin needed to be "tucked in," while his cheekbones were not prominent enough. He admitted to a number of difficulties in his current life. His employment history included many jobs in which, despite some success, he soon became dissatisfied, lost interest and resigned. He described himself as popular with women, but none of his relationships appeared to be significant. His girlfriends compared unfavorably with his mother, whom he idolized. He entertained unrealistic fantaasizes of attaining fame and stardom. He was impatient to have more surgery, which he believed would bring these hopes to fruition quickly.

The Surgery Addict

The insatiable patient should not be confused with the surgery addict. The surgery addict seeks repeated but different surgeries in an unending quest for physical self-improvement by surgical means. Appearance management is an ongoing project in much the same way that homeowners undertake successive remodeling projects on a house. As with any addiction, getting surgery takes on the flavor of a compulsion that provides at least temporary anxiety reduction. A good example is that of a woman who, over a period of about ten years, had first a breast reduction, then a tummy tuck, a nose operation, a face-lift, and then liposuction of her thighs. She was already planning to return for another face-lift and more liposuction. She talked openly and enthusiastically of her many surgeries and her plans for more. Not only did she declare great satisfaction with her results, but she was also ready to go back for more "in a minute." Often the surgery addict feels she is fighting a war of attrition with her looks. This was the case for "Barbara."

Although Barbara claimed her age was 48, she was actually 54. Despite her blonde hair, endless array of skin creams, and frequent shopping trips for new clothes, Barbara was having difficulty holding her marriage together. Her husband (age 55) was a wealthy businessman who traveled around the world and had casual affairs whenever he could. He had a habit of seducing Barbara's friends and then having them all together for lavish parties. Barbara had had her face lifted twice in attempts to remain youthful, and while these interventions were technically successful, they never altered her worried and guilty manner. She was very attached to her plastic surgeon, always bringing flowers for his secretary and returning regularly to have the state of her face checked by him. Barbara did her best to maintain the appearance of a good marriage, and she was generally known as a perfect hostess and long-suffering wife. However, her quiet unhappiness persisted. She felt that the creases that were removed from her face helped her look younger and conceal her inner misery. She felt she could not give up this approach to manage her life.

Perhaps the most bizarre case of a surgery addict is that of a 46-year-old French performance artist named Orlan. The *San Francisco Chronicle* reported that after nine operations on her face, she is still not finished.[34] According to the newspaper report, Orlan has dedicated her body to art. "She says she wants to look like a composite of prominent women in art and mythology, including the Mona Lisa, Venus and Diana." Her quest is not for ideal beauty, which is evident from the results. Her unnaturally high forehead with jutting eyebrows is topped with a dark-blue tuft of hair, and she looks to most observers as if something had gone drastically wrong in her surgery. She has had silicone implants over each eyebrow and in her cheeks, as well as a prosthetic put in her chin. "What I want is a complete transformation—to have the old image erased. At the end of all the operations, I'm going to get a new name and change my identity completely," says Orlan, whose original name was Mireille Porte.

This case may also be the first *folie a deux*—an induced psychotic disorder in which two people share a similar delusional system—in the annals of cosmetic surgery. (Technically, this situation is probably a case of *folie imposée*—in which there is one dominant delusional person and a second, more submissive person who absorbs the more dominant person's delusion.) Orlan convinced Dr. Marjorie Cramer, a New York plastic surgeon, that her motivation for surgery was a legitimate aesthetic expression and even got Dr. Cramer to wave her fee in the name of art. Perhaps Orlan and Dr. Cramer are not so crazy after all, though—they sell videos of the operations as well as pieces of her preserved flesh. It remains to be seen if Orlan will ultimately be satisfied when their artwork is finished.

Survivors of Abuse and Persons with an Eating Disorder

Some who seek cosmetic surgery have special issues. According to one study, some women with a history of childhood sexual abuse have greater dislike for their bodies than do those who have not suffered such abuse.[35] There is some evidence that abuse survivors are more likely to seek cosmetic surgery. Rarely are surgeons made aware of a history of abuse, even though it severely damages the survivor's body image. Surgery can trigger terrifying recall and flashbacks of prior abuse, as well as fears that the surgeon or the surgery would be abusive.

Likewise, those with an eating disorder may be more likely to want surgery.[36] (Two types of eating disorders are currently recognized. Anorexia involves the restriction of food and caloric intake and the consequent reduction of body weight to subsequentially below normal and often to a life-threatening level. Bulimia involves alternating binge eating and purging— compensation by vomiting or use of laxatives or excessive exercise. Bulimics are usually of normal weight. Both anorexics and bulimics share a morbid fear of fatness and body image disturbance.) In particular, requests for liposuction appear to be associated with a high incidence of eating disorders. Surgery serves to temporarily diminish the depression that underlies an eating disorder, but the dissatisfaction with the appearance of the body returns despite apparently satisfactory results from surgery. When childhood sexual abuse or an eating disorder exists, the sufferer should check with a therapist trained in such issues to better understand how the desire for cosmetic surgery may be related to either of these issues and to assist the patient, should any untoward emotions arise in conjunction with the surgery.[37]

Summary

More and more people of all ages and ethnic backgrounds, both men and women, are seeking cosmetic surgery. Women continue to be the predominant seekers, and fewer social sanctions against such surgery exist for them. Cosmetic surgery can often help children and teens develop more self-confidence and avoid rejection by peers, but should not be undertaken lightly. Some distress about appearance, especially for teens, is normal and usually does not warrant a trip to the surgeon. Fewer and fewer minorities are seeking cosmetic surgery to change their ethnic features. As their economic status rises, minorities in the United States generally seek cosmetic surgery to enhance their appearance while preserving their racial and ethnic identity. Because of the special problems minorities can face with scarring and pigmentation changes, it is especially important for them to seek out surgeons who are specially trained in working with minorities. Although most people who seek surgery are "normal" and healthy emotionally, some who want surgery are psychiatrically impaired. The kinds of emotional problems that may lead some people to seek cosmetic surgery include having severe body image disturbance, having a personality disorder, or being psychotic or delusional. Finally, survivors of childhood sexual abuse or those who suffer from an eating disorder should discuss their desire for cosmetic surgery with a therapist to avoid difficult psychological reactions to surgery.

6

Okay, Schedule Me

My first encounter with a plastic surgeon was in 1982. A good friend referred me to Dr. K. to have a prominent scar on my left cheek revised. The scar had been inflicted by a dog bite, and Dr. K. performed a Z-plasty—a special procedure that makes a scar less visible by altering its direction. Not long after, I started going to Dr. K. for collagen injections for the treatment of fine wrinkles. Even though Dr. K. used a very fine syringe to inject the collagen into the depressions of the wrinkles and stretched the skin while doing so to minimize discomfort, the injections were incredibly painful. I imagined that having my finger nails pulled out one at a time couldn't be worse. The injection sites were red and puffy for a day, and for a few days a little raised ridge was visible where the wrinkle depression had been. Soon my face returned to normal, only to gradually develop those same wrinkles again as the collagen was absorbed by my body. I returned to Dr. K. every three or four months to repeat the procedure. By the time I started thinking about getting a face-lift in 1990, Dr. K. had announced his retirement, and I had to find another plastic surgeon.

I started gathering information by calling names I found in ads or in the phone book. "Come in and look at our before-and-after pictures," suggested one doctor's nurse I reached. Everyone offered to send me brochures explaining various cosmetic procedures and invited me to come for a consultation, the cost of which would be applied to an operation if I chose to proceed. I was confronted with a bewildering array of credentials and names of organizations to which a particular surgeon belonged. "Be sure the one you pick is 'board certified' and has lots of experience," said one doctor's receptionist on the telephone. Certified by whom? For what? What is the difference between "Board Certified in Plastic Surgery" and "Board Certified Plastic Surgeon?" How much experience is enough? What do the initials "F.A.C.S." after a surgeon's name mean? Should I care? Then I met a woman who had had a face-lift and was pleased with her surgeon and her results. She showed me her before-and-after pictures and told me about her surgeon's impressive credentials. I telephoned his office for a consultation the next day.

Upon my arrival in the doctor's waiting room, a tall, slender, attractive blond woman, dressed tastefully in a fashionable outfit, greeted me. She was the doctor's nurse. I was surprised; she looked more like a model than a nurse. She showed me into a small room with a video monitor. "We think it's helpful for our patients to understand more about cosmetic surgery. After you watch this video, the doctor will see you." On a low coffee table were copies of articles on the doctor's work that had been published in *Vogue* and *Newsweek* and in local newspapers.

Later I was directed to Dr. A.'s office, which was large and furnished with expensively upholstered furniture and Oriental artifacts. I was seated in front of a large, mahogany desk, which was very neat with a small brass lamp on one side. Dr. A. strode into the office and extended his hand to me. What an imposing presence. He was very tall, with white hair, and seemed to be in his late 50s or early 60s. The consultation began with what seemed to be small talk. How old was I? Was I married? How were things with me? How long had I been thinking of getting a face-lift? What did I hope the surgery would do for me? Little did I realize that these questions were intended to elicit information that would help him decide whether I was psychologically a good candidate for surgery. The focus changed to what could be done. He explained that in addition to the SMAS procedure, a forehead lift and eyelid surgery, as well as liposuction under the chin, were needed to produce the best possible results. "Of course, as with any surgery, there are risks," he continued. I don't remember any of the rest of this conversation, but I do remember signing a form saying that the doctor had discussed risks of the operation with me. At some point, I asked about the cost. "I don't talk about that, but I can tell you, I'm very expensive. My nurse will discuss money issues with you."

The nurse/model took me to a different room, and we sat down at a round table with a view of a lovely garden. Dr. A. had written out for her the various procedures he had recommended for me. She completed a form indicating each procedure to be performed and the total surgical fee, which included the doctor's fee for consultation, pre-operative examination, pre- and post-operative photographs, and all post-operative visits. That total was $13,750. The additional costs of the operating and recovery rooms (located in the surgeon's facilities), the anesthesiologist, the guest room in the hospital across the street, and incidentals brought the grand total to $15,595. (Fees for cosmetic surgery operations vary considerably from surgeon to surgeon depending on reputation and locality.) The figure was nearly double what I had expected. "The doctor's operating schedule fills up quickly, and if you want a particular date, you really should schedule soon. To get your date on the calendar, we'll need a refundable deposit of $1,350 now. The balance must be received three weeks before the scheduled operation date."

"Good grief! I could buy a small car for the cost of this operation, but at least I could finance a car," I thought to myself. (Although it is almost universal to collect fees in advance, some surgeons do provide information on financing.) "I could shop around for a lower fee, but do I want to trust my face to a bargain basement surgeon?" My thoughts continued, "I could make the appointment now so I get the date I want, and I can cancel later if necessary. That way I can have time to think about this."

"Okay, schedule me for October 9." As I left the doctor's offices, I felt heavy of heart. How could I afford to spend so much money on this kind of thing? Yet, not to go ahead with the face-lift I had said for so many years I would get seemed unthinkable. I'd already invested a lot of time and energy getting information and telling my friends I was going to do this. How could I retreat now? I didn't realize it then, but I was in the "action" stage of change.

The Stages of Change

Although not specific to cosmetic surgery, there is research that suggests how people undertake self-improvement and change.[1] If we apply this model of change, undergoing a cosmetic surgery operation can be seen as the end result of a series of self-change stages, each characterized by a particular way of thinking that impacts decision making and behavior. In the first or *precontemplation* stage, little thought is given to obtaining cosmetic surgery and no intention exists to do so in the foreseeable future. Young people and those who do not perceive themselves as having an important or changeable deficit in appearance are in this stage.

When aging begins to affect appearance or when self-consciousness about a body part or feature becomes painful, the person suffering these effects begins to think seriously about how to overcome the problem. In this *contemplation* stage, there is not yet a commitment to action. Both the pros and cons of various solutions, which may include having cosmetic surgery, are about equally considered. A prospective patient struggles with the positive rewards of cosmetic surgery—looking and feeling better about oneself—and the costs in terms of time, money, physical pain, and the possibly negative opinions of others for considering such action.

Once the intention to take action is formed, a person enters the *preparation* stage. She takes certain steps toward the goal of obtaining surgery—noticing and reading articles in magazines and newspapers about cosmetic surgery, reading brochures and books on the subject, and soliciting the opinions of family, friends, and acquaintances. At some point, she may contact a plastic surgeon for a consultation. These small steps prepare her for the ultimate step—making the commitment to undergo an operation.

During the preparation stage, there is a shift in thinking about the balance of pros and cons of surgery. The prospective patient begins to attend selectively to information that supports one or the other points of view. If cons begin to outweigh pros, further action is discontinued, and the decision is made not to seek surgery, at least at this time. With increasing aging or self-consciousness, the balance may shift again and initiate renewed action. Often by the time a person goes to the doctor's office for a consultation, she is already focusing more on the pros. Information that argues against surgery is likely to be dismissed, distorted, or denied. At this point, a prospective patient does not "hear" the doctor's discussion of risks or physical trauma, or she forgets it quickly. If the pros increasingly outweigh the cons in her mind, and if she decides she likes and trusts this doctor and can afford the cost, she moves into the next stage.

The *action* stage is when she makes the commitment to have surgery and says, "Okay, schedule me." Her thinking now focuses on what needs to be done in preparation for surgery. Although it is possible to slip back into a previous stage and experience a resurgence of doubts (some patients who schedule operations cancel without rescheduling), the thinking of a person in the action stage is geared to screen out doubts and focus on action that supports the decision.

The Decision-Making Process

Feminist writers and others deplore the media for promoting the "beauty myth" and planting the seeds of self-rejection. The ideal female body as seen in the media is young, thin, athletic, and busty, and unattainable by most real women. Women can come to believe that some aspect of their bodies is ugly and repulsive, setting the stage for eating disorders, depression, and possibly an insatiable appetite for cosmetic surgery.

While it is true that the media promotes certain unrealistic ideals, the media is also a major source of information on health for most people, and has significant potential for shaping and changing attitudes.[2] A 1990 Times Mirror study reported in *Advertising Age* found that television is the preferred news source of American women.[3] TV is also the most cited source of health information, followed by newspapers, women's magazines, news magazines, and radio.[4] The media has had an impact on American women in a variety of health issues, including pregnancy, premenstrual syndrome, toxic shock, and menopause. At times, the treatment of these issues has been distorted, negative, confusing, misleading, and alarming.[5] The coverage is almost always sensationalist. Decision making based on bad information is necessarily poor.

A few years ago the media gave a lot of attention to the safety of breast implants. This was partly prompted by Food and Drug Administration (FDA) when they issued a voluntary moratorium on January 6, 1992 on silicone gel breast implants because of reports of ruptured silicone "bleeding" through the envelope, and posing serious health risks, such as cancer and autoimmune disorders. The FDA later banned the sale of silicone implants, despite a published report from the American Medical Association (AMA) that the anxiety over breast implants "is not warranted based on current scientific evidence." The AMA reported that "no clinical data are available that definitively prove that an increased incidence of breast cancer or any other type of cancer is associated with silicone gel breast implants." It also dismissed any connection between silicone gel breast implants and autoimmune disorders. Nevertheless, television "magazine shows" continued the controversy, often by airing horrific stories told by women whose implants had ruptured, allowing silicone to migrate to other parts of the body and cause damage. Magazines also continued to print stories about the aftereffects of silicone implants, including arthritis-like joint pain, fatigue, and hardening of the breasts.

Indeed, there was no shortage of anecdotal stories about the dangers of silicone. The case of Barbara, a 31-year-old journalist who had her breasts enlarged in 1976, was reported in *Reader's Digest*.[6] "The doctor said it was a safe and simple thing to do, like permanent-waving my hair," she recalled. Within months, her breasts began to harden. Eventually she returned to the surgeon, who diagnosed the problem as "just scar tissue" and indicated it could be easily fixed. He then squeezed her breast to break up the scar tissue. The procedure was painful, and she was given no sedation. The next day, she noticed a knot inside her breast. The implant had ruptured and the silicone had leaked. Barbara returned to the doctor, who replaced the implant. Soon, Barbara began to feel weak and short of breath. She developed stiffness and pain in her shoulders, hips, legs, wrists, and ankles. She noticed she was losing some of her hair, and experiencing chills and fever. Eventually she was diagnosed as suffering from an autoimmune-like disease that some doctors believed was brought on by the silicone leakage. Her condition may be progressive and incurable.

Janet van Winkle, 49, of Kirkwood, Missouri, told her story in *First for Women* magazine.[7] She too got her first silicone implants in 1976. In 1982 she developed breast cancer, and doctors removed both breasts. After her double mastectomy, she had breast reconstruction with a new set of silicone implants. Two years later she returned for the first of six operations to repair and replace ruptured and leaking implants. Subsequently, she developed a host of medical problems. "I have silicone in my lungs," she says. "I have nerve damage. I can't stand up for long periods of time. If I had to get dressed and go to work every day, I couldn't do it." Although bedridden most of the time, in 1990 she founded American Silicone Implant Survivors (314-821-0115), a self-help group for those who have suffered problems.

Research about the media's reporting of the safety of silicone gel breast implants, as well as breast augmentation and reconstruction procedures, found that most women took the information seriously.[8] Women who had, or were thinking of having, elective breast augmentation surgery were more likely to believe what they heard in the media than those who needed breast reconstruction because of disease. After the FDA moratorium, a majority of women (about 60 percent) became convinced of the dangers of silicone leakage and the risks related to breast surgery. Satisfaction with the decision to have implants changed from 98 percent before the moratorium to 71 percent for augmentation patients and 79 percent for reconstruction patients. Fewer women sought such surgery after this media attention, and they were less likely to believe plastic surgeons. A survey of 500 women conducted by ASPRS in February of 1992 suggested that media coverage may have undermined surgeons as a credible source of information, at least for breast implants.[9]

Today, the silicone scare has faded from media coverage and from the minds of many women. Women's magazines regularly carry articles on various aspects of cosmetic surgery, and newspapers report on new developments. One source of information, however, remains relatively untapped. Talking to friends and others who have had cosmetic surgery can be very helpful, but often is not done. Despite the increasing acceptance and popularity of cosmetic surgery, there are still taboos. Unlike dieting, having cosmetic surgery is not yet a casual topic of conversation at cocktail parties. Even so, a surprising number of people might admit to having had cosmetic surgery or to wanting to do so. Talking with someone who has gone through the same operation gives the opportunity to ask questions and voice fears in a way that is different from talking to the doctor.

The Consultation

The surgeon and the patient have different aims in the initial consultation. The surgeon needs to determine whether it is reasonably possible to provide the result a prospective patient wants from surgery. For this reason it is important that she be able to articulate what she expects. Simply saying "I want to look better" does not give the surgeon enough information. The patient may think the doctor is an expert who will determine on his own what to do and recommend it but, in fact, what the doctor thinks would be an improvement and what the patient thinks may not coincide. The doctor needs to know what feature the patient is dissatisfied with and how the patient wants it to look. Once the patient provides the surgeon with her view of the problem, the doctor can determine which procedures will be necessary to achieve a solution. Sometimes what the patient wants as the result of surgery cannot be achieved. The patient's anatomy won't permit it. For example, little can be done to alter the appearance of deep set eyes with prominent, bony rims. The surgeon must evaluate not only what the patient wants but whether the requested change is possible.

Sometimes surgeons recommend more procedures and greater change than their patients initially had in mind. Surgeons are guided by their own ideas of what constitutes a good result and can at times be swept away by possibilities. Often patients are hesitant to disagree, believing that the doctor knows best. For their own mental health and to protect the doctor/patient relationship from strain, patients should ask for a more modest or incremental approach to change if what the doctor suggests doesn't feel comfortable.

In addition, the surgeon needs to determine if this patient is psychologically appropriate for surgery. The principle goal of aesthetic surgery is the emotional satisfaction of the patient, and if this cannot be reasonably achieved, surgery should be deferred or denied. Patient satisfaction with results depends on a number of factors, the most important of which is whether the patient's expectations for surgery are realistic. A patient who expects surgery to fix other problems in life or relieve emotional distress related to other issues has unrealistic expectations for what surgery can do.

The possiblity of patient dissatisfaction can raise questions about the appropriateness of surgery. A patient who has a very minimal defect in appearance but who is excessively concerned or distressed about it should be a danger signal to the surgeon. Patients who want surgery primarily to satisfy someone else, or who hope surgery will fix feelings of sexual inadequacy, are not good candidates. People who are visibly depressed or paranoid can develop post-operative problems. When a patient praises the surgeon excessively and denigrates another, especially if the results of the previous surgery are objectively acceptable, the surgeon is likely to be reluctant to operate. Patients who are rude, demanding, obsessive, indecisive, or who don't tell the whole truth may be rejected. Those who are hesitant to undress or who refuse to have pictures taken signal problems as well. The socially prominent or famous person may expect special treatment that is inappropriate. Surgery may be contraindicated for the person who is in therapy but who hasn't gotten the approval of her therapist and won't agree to allow the surgeon to talk to the therapist.

Surgeons should evaluate the patient's degree of self-consciousness. Patients who are only slightly self-conscious are more at risk for post-operative distress than those who are highly self-conscious. They need to fully understand the limitations and risks of surgery, and may need additional pre-operative consultations to digest the implications of surgery. In most cases, patients who are not at all self-conscious about a presumed defect should not be operated on, although others who are not especially self-conscious may request surgery for professional reasons.

If it appears that surgery can correct the perceived defect, and if the patient's expectations for surgery and her psychological status indicate that she is appropriate for surgery, the surgeon will go on to discuss what procedures are needed to achieve the desired results. At this point, he should also discuss the risks and complications that can occur and have the patient sign a form indicating that this discussion took place. The purpose of this is both to protect the surgeon from accusations he did not fully inform the patient and to call the patient's attention to the importance of taking the potential risks and complications of surgery seriously. The surgeon also attempts to allay the patient's anxiety and support her decision to proceed with surgery.

If the decision is made to proceed, the surgeon will discuss the type of anesthesia to be used—local or general—and accompanying risk that may be incurred. Local anesthesia involves the injection of a drug into the area to be operated on, causing local numbness. Although some drowsiness can occur, patients are awake and aware, but feel nothing during the operation. Pressure or pulling may be felt, but no pain. Patients under a local may or may not remember what their experiences were during the operation. For very minor operations under local anesthesia, no intravenous line or complicated monitoring is required. More involved and prolonged procedures, such as face-lifts, are frequently done under general anesthesia, which carries greater risks. The patient is asleep for the entire operation and surgery is painless. The services of an anesthesiologist are required, which raises the cost of the operation. In addition, there is an increased possibility of bruising, the risk of infection, and more problems during recovery, including possible nausea, vomiting, and prolonged drowsiness.

The Patient's Agenda

By the time the patient goes for a consultation, her mind is largely made up, and she is selectively attending to information that will support her decision for surgery. Even though she is presumably there to get the surgeon's input on what can be done to fix the perceived defect, in fact she has her own hidden agenda and is responding to more subtle clues. "Do I like this doctor? Can I trust him? Is his staff nice? Do I feel comfortable here?" The surgeon's credentials may or may not be heavily weighed at this point. "How does the doctor see my problem? What can be done to fix it? How long will it take? How much will it cost? Can I afford it? How much time off do I need? How can I arrange for it? With these questions crowding her mind, there is little wonder that she doesn't remember the discussion on risks and complications.

Assessing the Doctor's Qualifications

The greater acceptance and continued growth of cosmetic surgery among the general public has encouraged more and more doctors to enter this field. The rush for the scalpel has come about because cosmetic surgery provides a lucrative profit in an otherwise complicated health-care payment system. As the reimbursed costs of medical procedures shrink, and doctors are paid sometimes as little as 30 cents on the dollar for their services, a cosmetic surgery practice looks increasingly attractive. Patients choose cosmetic surgery—not insurance companies who don't reimburse for elective procedures—and patients pay all costs in cash, in advance. Cosmetic surgeons get 100 cents on the dollar. No wonder wanna-be plastic surgeons are hanging out their uncredentialed shingles, and the public doesn't understand the difference.

Several years ago, an investigation by the House Small Business Subcommittee on Regulation found that far too much cosmetic surgery was being done by doctors who had no special training in the field. These doctors operate in outpatient offices that are often not equipped to deal with emergencies. Legally, anyone with a medical license can perform any operation, whether trained in that procedure or not. Doctors who may have only had a short seminar at a tropical resort are opening shop as cosmetic surgeons. They need answer to no one. Major surgery is done in hospitals, where doctors aren't allowed to perform procedures they aren't qualified to do. Cosmetic surgery is mostly performed in private outpatient clinics, away from the watchful eyes of review boards or peers. There are no minimum standards for outpatient clinics, and no guarantees that they are well staffed or well equipped.

The subcommittee investigation found that these "cosmetic surgeons" often used deceptive ads mentioning false or meaningless credentials, such as fellowships in medical societies that required only the payment of dues. Some ads included the words "board certified," when the doctor was certified in a specialty having little to do with the advertised cosmetic procedures. Glossy ads made the surgery seem fast and affordable, and glorified promises attempted to persuade patients that the surgeons were qualified to perform anything from a chemical peel to a tummy tuck.

A *Glamour* magazine article tells the story of Dona, a professional model who responded to an advertisement in a local city magazine.[10] "Be a Knockout!" the ad promised, picturing a trim, well-toned model, and listing procedures from nose sculpting to liposuction to breast implants. The ad indicated that procedures were performed by "acknowledged specialists in our state-of-the-art facility." The consultation was more like a bargaining session, with the doctor dropping the price for a breast augmentation from $4,000, the going rate at the time, to $1,500. Several days after her surgery, Dona's breasts began to harden, and she was alarmed to find that one breast was significantly higher than the other. The doctor assured her they would "even themselves out," but they didn't. Eventually Dona found another surgeon who was willing to repair the botched job, though it cost her $4,000 more.

An important distinction must be made between a "cosmetic surgeon" and a "plastic surgeon." A cosmetic surgeon is a specialist in surgical procedures that enhance appearance, such as face-lifts and breast augmentation. A plastic surgeon is trained in both cosmetic and reconstructive surgery, such as hand surgery, skin grafts, cleft palate repair, and procedures that help patients to function better. In addition, plastic surgeons are trained in general surgery. They complete a minimum of three years residency in general surgery and two in plastic surgery. Many "cosmetic surgeons"—who may be anything from general practitioners to gynecologists—receive relatively little training before they open a cosmetic surgery practice.

Some physicians receive cosmetic surgery training as part of their training in a particular specialty. Ear, nose, and throat specialists are trained to do cosmetic surgery from the neck up. Ophthalmologists may be trained in cosmetic surgery of the eyes. Dermatologists are trained in procedures performed on the surface of the skin. General surgeons have extensive training in breast surgery, but little training in cosmetic breast surgery or body contouring. These physicians may become "board certified" by a board related to their specialty.

When a physician indicates he or she is "board certified," the important question to ask is, "Which board?" A mind-boggling number of medical organizations have evolved that provide certification of one kind or another. Different boards have different qualifications and standards for potential candidates. Some of these certifications are meaningful, and others are not. The designation "board certified plastic surgeon" usually means that the surgeon wishes to be regarded as a plastic surgeon when he has been trained in another field.

A physician who is "board certified in plastic surgery" has been certified by the American Board of Plastic Surgery, the official examining board for plastic surgeons. Holders of this certification are qualified to perform reconstructive and cosmetic surgery. Similarly, ophthalmologists can obtain board certification to do cosmetic surgery on eyelids, dermatologists on skin procedures, and otolaryngologists on the head and neck. These latter specialists would not be board certified in plastic surgery without the training and experience designated by the American Board of Plastic Surgery.

Most plastic surgeons argue that only those physicians who are certified by boards recognized by the American Board of Medical Specialties (ABMS) should be doing cosmetic surgery. (The Appendix gives a list of boards recognized by the ABMS, as well as a list of self-designated boards not recognized by the ABMS.) The American Board of Plastic Surgery, which is recognized by the ABMS, is the only board that certifies plastic surgeons. The candidates must complete thousands of hours of training before performing plastic surgery and provide evidence of competency in the particular type of cosmetic surgery for which certification is sought.

The *Directory of Medical Specialists,* which may be found in many public libraries, lists the names of surgeons who are board certified for particular procedures. A similar reference is the *Compendium of Certified Medical Specialists,* which is kept up to date by the ABMS. It is also possible to call the ABMS, at 1-800-776-2378, to check a doctor's credentials. Although board certification is not a guarantee, it is one piece of evidence toward evaluating a surgeon. If the ABMS does not recognize the board providing the certification, it is probably a self-designated board which has not subjected itself to peer evaluation. Certifications from such organizations are probably meaningless.

In addition to advocating cosmetic surgery certification only by boards recognized by the ABMS, most plastic surgeons also argue that physicians should only perform procedures in the specialty for which they have been certified. Thus a certified otolaryngologist should only do surgery on the neck and above, not on breasts or other parts of the body. Physicians with other surgical specialties often regard this as an attempt by plastic surgeons to keep the lucrative cosmetic surgery market to themselves. Some of these physicians have set up their own organizations in order to legitimize their practices. One of these is the American Board of Cosmetic Surgery. To belong, the physician must be evaluated by his peers and pass an examination, but a surgical residency is not required. For other organizations, all that may be required to belong is the payment of a few hundred dollars.

Patients have been hurt by physicians holding themselves out as "board certified" by bogus organizations. A case was reported of a young Los Angeles man who wanted his nose straightened.[11] The doctor he consulted claimed to be a "board certified specialist in cosmetic surgery." Four operations later, the man had lost most of his nose. It took ten more operations by another surgeon and over $50,000 to reconstruct some semblance of normalcy. His cosmetic surgeon turned out to be a general practitioner with no formal training in plastic surgery.

Another woman, who was a registered nurse, went to a "board certified cosmetic surgeon" who listed breast surgery as one of his specialities.[12] As soon as the bandages came off, she noticed that her breasts were deformed. The implants had been put in the wrong place, and one stuck out below the nipple. She spent over $20,000 on reconstructive surgeries with another doctor and had to live with a deformity for two years. It turned out that the first doctor misrepresented himself as a qualified surgeon. His training consisted of a three-day seminar in the Bahamas.

Also the number of letters following a physicians name is not an indicator of any particular expertise in plastic surgery. For example, "F.A.C.S." stands for fellow of the American College of Surgeons. This is certainly a prestigious organization, but its main focus is educational and political. This designation in no way guarantees that the surgeon is qualified to do plastic surgery or any particular cosmetic technique. Prospective patients should not be impressed because of multiple letters following a doctor's name, nor simply by the words, "board certified." More information is needed to determine a surgeon's qualifications.

Qualifying a Surgeon

1. Ask the doctor directly if he is board certified and by which board.

2. If the doctor is certified in a particular area of the body, is the procedure you're considering in that area of specialty? If yes, ask for the name and number of the certifying organization so you can find out

their requirements for certification. (If they don't require a residency, beware.) If the doctor is not certified to operate on the area you want changed, consider looking for another surgeon.

3. Check the doctor's credentials. Call the American Board of Medical Specialties at 1-800-776-2378, or check your local library for either the *Directory of Medical Specialists* or the *Compendium of Certified Medical Specialists* to see if he is listed. Also check the certificates on the doctor's wall to see what certifications are displayed.

4. Ask the doctor about his experience. How many times has he performed the procedure you want done? Choose someone who has done it hundreds, if not thousands, of times.

5. Ask if the doctor is on the staff of a major hospital. Call the hospital and ask if he has privileges in the hospital to perform the specific procedure you desire—even if your surgery is to be done in his office or clinic.

6. If the surgery will be done in the doctor's outpatient clinic or surgical center, ask if the clinic or center is accredited and if an experienced anesthetist will be used.

7. Ask the doctor to provide you with the names and phone numbers of former patients who had the same procedure so you can talk to them about their experience. Doctors feel an obligation to protect the privacy of their patients, but they should be able to provide some contacts.

8. Be wary of doctors who use slick advertising or who promise terrific results.

9. Be wary of doctors who don't ask about your motivations and expectations for surgery, who gloss over risks and complications, or who fail to discuss how the operation might affect you emotionally.

10. Be wary of doctors who fail to take a medical history or don't do a thorough physical examination beforehand.

Physical Preparation for Surgery

Once doctor and patient agree about what needs to be done for the desired surgical result and the decision to proceed is made, they must coordinate to schedule a date for surgery. It may be several months before there is an opening in the surgeon's schedule, and the patient needs time to prepare. Patients need to arrange time off from work or assistance at home. Depending on the operation, most people need at least ten days of rest and recovery before they have enough energy to return to their regular activities. Facial surgery requires even longer—usually about three weeks to look presentable. Even then, it is unlikely that all swelling and bruising will be gone, and makeup will probably be needed to cover up bruises.

At some point the doctor will discuss how to prepare for surgery. For two weeks before surgery, no aspirin or aspirin derivatives should be used, nor vitamin E, or estrogen. Ideally, the patient should be in the best possible health before surgery. Patients who are overweight should try to slim down. If significant weight is lost after surgery, the post-operative results may not be as satisfactory. Smokers should quit smoking at once if possible, or at least two weeks before surgery. Not only does smoking create small wrinkles around the mouth, nicotine reduces blood flow to the skin. Some surgeons won't do face-lifts on smokers because the poor circulation from smoking increases the chance of skin loss behind the ears and elsewhere. Alcohol consumption also should be curtailed. Excessive alcohol use increases risk from surgery, and use afterwards contributes to fluid retention (edema) and swelling of the skin. Periodic, recurring episodes of edema can cause the skin to stretch and sag, especially around the eyes.

After the decision is made to proceed, and before the operation takes place, the surgeon should take a complete medical history and do a thorough physical exam to be sure the patient's physical health is adequate. It is important that the patient let the surgeon know about any physical problems so that the doctor can anticipate and work around the obstacles such problems may pose. Rarely do physical problems prevent surgery.

Psychological Preparation for Surgery

Once the decision to go ahead with surgery has been made and a date scheduled, patients have their own ways of getting ready, which may or may not be helpful.

> *Paulette.* Paulette, whose father was a well-respected cancer specialist, considered herself to be something of an expert in herbal and Chinese medicine. Her preparation for surgery included consuming daily potions of herbs she concocted to prepare herself for the trauma any surgery brings, and she meditated daily to minimize any emotional trauma. In the several weeks before her surgery, she did her yoga exercises, and got regular, full-body massages.

> *Jackie.* Jackie did what she knew worked; she continued her dedicated pursuit of physical fitness at the gym. She increased her workouts, with special attention to her pectoral muscles. Although she had always been careful to avoid fats in her diet, she began paying particular attention to eating right.

Helen. Helen rented a furnished apartment, which she stocked with books to read and videos to watch during recovery. Her plan was to recover alone, out of sight of her husband and children, until she felt ready to present her new self.

How prospective patients prepare for surgery influences how well they cope with recovery. Making positive changes such as losing weight, getting physically fit, quitting smoking, and minimizing stress are likely to help. Knowing what to expect, and being mentally, as well as physically, prepared to cope are also important.

Research clearly shows that patients who are psychologically prepared reap significant benefits.[13] How best to prepare is just beginning to be understood. The most effective components in an adequate preparation for surgery include getting information about sensory effects, and adopting behavioral and cognitive coping methods.[14] When patients are informed about the physical sensations that are likely to accompany surgery, such as feeling pressure, pulling, or tingling, or smelling an odor or hearing a sound if under a local, they are less likely to become anxious. Visiting and viewing the operating room beforehand can also help allay anxiety. Knowing what to expect during recovery helps patients put their sensations and feelings into perspective. When forewarned that they may initially feel euphoric and then become depressed, but that eventually they will return to normal, they are better able to cope. Patients who have been taught to use relaxation, guided imagery, or distraction techniques are better able to manage anxiety and discomfort. A good attitude and using coping self-talk is also helpful. The use of such techniques has been shown to reduce negative feelings, pain, the need for pain medication, and length of stay in the hospital.

In getting ready psychologically for surgery, patients need to understand and prepare for the "Four Ds" that characterize the aftermath of surgery—dependency, dysphoria (feeling unhappy), denial, and direction.[15] After surgery, the patient comes home weak, weary, and unsure of herself. Initially she is able to stay in bed or at home and rest, without having to immediately take up her usual chores. Often someone is there to take care of her, at least for the first few days. It feels good to be helped, and consciously or unconsciously, the patient may encourage more of it, even when it is no longer required. It may be hard to find the energy to get going again, and a certain amount of dependency on others may be fostered.

Energy loss at this time is also related to negative emotions, usually depressed feelings. Without energy, thoughts become increasingly negative. The hallmark thoughts of depression are, "It's me. It affects everything I do. It's never going to change." Interpretations of events turn sour and pessimistic. Awareness of the possibility of negativity and depression help prepare the patient to be more positive.

Denial as a psychological defense mechanism, used judiciously, isn't always bad. Putting aside thoughts about bruising, swelling, and pain can be helpful. Staying busy, distracting oneself with other thoughts, or using guided imagery are some ways to avoid dwelling on the pain and discomfort.

Thinking about the future is important. A healthy person has direction, short- and long-term goals. Energy is needed to accomplish goals. The patient must get personal control over her energy, much like a long-distance runner trying to complete a marathon race. Running too fast will deplete energy. The key is to find a pace that will allow completion of the race. The patient in recovery from surgery needs to pace herself so that she doesn't run out of either physical or emotional energy.

Most of all, anxiety, depression, and other symptoms need to be placed in proper perspective. Planning ahead and knowing what to expect, preparing by learning to relax or using guided imagery, and creating a positive, coping attitude are indispensable approaches for getting ready for surgery.

Summary

By the time the patient gets to the surgeon's office for a consultation, she is more focused on the pros than the cons of getting surgery. As a result, her tendency is to screen out information about risks and complications and to focus on information that supports her desire for surgery. Too often, patients don't take the time, or make the effort, or don't know how to assess a doctor's qualifications. Patients have their own ways of preparing for surgery, but their actions may or may not help. There are effective techniques for preparing psychologically for surgery, and these include being forewarned about what to expect and being prepared to take coping actions.

It was 7:00 A.M., the time appointed for me to arrive at the doctor's office. The procedure would take place in the operating room that was part of his office. Afterwards I would be taken to the adjoining hospital for overnight observation.

My husband walked with me down the quiet, empty hall. I wore the new warm-ups I had purchased for the occasion, white nylon with purple, black, and blue trim over the shoulders. The significance of the colors didn't register at the time. I had a hard time finding a T-shirt that buttoned; I was told not to wear anything that had to go over my head. We entered the doctor's waiting room. The lamps on the end tables cast a soft glow on the expensive furnishings. It felt like evening and I was entering someone's home. In a hushed tone, one of the doctor's nurses, the one who dressed and looked like a fashion model, led me down the hall to a small examining room. The knot in the pit of my stomach was getting tighter.

"How are you?" asked the blue-robed nurse as she came into the room.

"Not too good. I'm terribly nervous."

"That's okay. We have some Valium to relax you. By the time we finish taking your 'before' pictures, you'll start feeling better."

After changing into a hospital gown, I said good-bye to my husband, and the nurses escorted me down the hall to the operating room. By this time, and with the help of the Valium, I was carrying on a friendly, if slightly tipsy, conversation with one of the nurses. My doctor and the anesthesiologist were waiting. While an intravenous line was being inserted into a vein in my left arm, I continued my one-sided conversation with the nurse. Then she said, "It's time now." The room bleached to white; then nothing.

7

What Have I Done?

"Hi honey, how are you feeling?"

I heard my husband's voice and felt someone take my hand. I couldn't see anything because of the cold compresses on my eyes. The head of the hospital bed and the section under my knees were elevated. Sometime earlier, after the surgery, I had been transferred from the operating room in my surgeon's office to the hospital across the street, where I was to stay overnight. A nurse was with me to change my compresses and administer pain medication. The operation had taken some six hours. I didn't know what time it was, but I sensed it must be evening.

"Tell the doctor the bandages are too tight," I whispered. It felt as though a tight strap had been cinched under my chin and over the top of my head. Bandages encircled my entire head and neck, leaving only my face uncovered, except for the compresses on my eyes.

I felt my husband touch the bandages around my face and head.

"Honey, the bandages are very loose," he said softly.

"No, no. They're too tight," I pleaded. He squeezed my hand gently. My mind seemed to stagger. How could the bandages be loose and feel so tight? Slowly it began to dawn on me, it wasn't the bandages. It was me. Good God, what have I done?

After he left, I dozed back to sleep, awakening briefly each time the nurse changed the compresses. Somewhere in the night, the pain sharpened, and a severe headache developed.

"Could I please have something for the pain?" I asked the nurse. My doctor had assured me that pain medication would be available.

"It's not time yet," said the nurse. "We have to wait another hour."

Another hour? In a few minutes, I tried again. "Please, it hurts a lot."

"I'm sorry, but we have to wait." Despite the sympathy in her voice, she apparently had a timetable for dispensing the medication, and she intended to follow it.

A little time passed, and again I pleaded, and again and again, until finally she relented.

"Okay. I'll give you half of a pain pill now, and the rest in half an hour when you're supposed to get it."

As the anesthesia wore off, I was less able to doze back to sleep. The cinched feeling under my chin made swallowing difficult and painful. I could hear the nurse turning the pages of a book or a magazine. Time crept by, and the pain seemed only slightly duller. That awful, cinched feeling was unrelenting. A flutter of panic arose from within me. No, I can't let that happen. Breathe. Just think about breathing. Think about anything—but the pain.

"I have to use the bathroom," I said. I heard the nurse stir from her chair and move toward me. She removed the compresses from my eyes and said, "Here, bring your legs to the edge of the bed." A wave of nausea hit me as I sat up. My eyes were swollen nearly shut, and I was unable to open them more than a crack. I could see a little sliver of light through the opening between my swollen eyelids, as if I were in a dark room and seeing light shining from underneath a closed door. I stood up, and the room began to swim. Breathe. Go slow. One step at a time.

With the nurse's support, I found my way to the bathroom. When I was finished, I moved toward the sink to wash my hands. Through the crack between my eyelids, I could see my hands. As I stood at the sink, I knew there was a mirror above it. I started to tilt my head back so I could see myself through the tiny opening between my lids.

"Don't look," said the nurse. "Please don't look." Her voice was soft, but her concern was evident. I knew she meant to protect me. I lowered my head without looking. I would wait a few days to see what I looked like. The nurse helped me back to bed.

The next morning, I was transported back to my doctor's office for a checkup before being released to go home. The stitches in my eyelids would come out in a few days. It would be a few weeks before the staples in my scalp were removed. I was told I could take a shower in 48 hours. It would be good to get home to my own bed.

Post-Operative Trauma

Cosmetic surgery is major surgery, and the recovery process is not insignificant. Wound healing is not a question of days or even weeks, but months in many cases.[1] According to a 1992 study, the level of post-operative trauma and distress is much greater than surgeons are aware of or patients are led to expect.[2] In this research, two groups of aftercare nurses who attended cosmetic surgery patients were studied. One group attended patients in recovery for an average of two to four days. Another group had contact with patients for at least one month and up to one year post-operatively. These nurses were asked about the percentage of their patients that experienced physical or mental anguish after cosmetic surgery. The longer nurses were in contact with patients, the more trauma and depression they observed. Those nurses who tended patients for only a few days following surgery reported that an average of 39 percent of their patients experienced some level of physical or mental trauma, and an average of 46 percent became depressed. Nurses who were in contact with patients longer indicated that an average of 94 percent of patients experienced such trauma and 97 percent developed depression at some point during the several months following surgery. The researcher concluded that patients were not prepared for the level of discomfort they would experience, nor for the temporary disfigurement that surgery inevitably produces and the resulting emotional difficulties.

Although serious, long-lasting emotional disturbances are believed to be rare, studies have confirmed that transient episodes of depression and anxiety occur during the days or weeks after surgery in over half of cosmetic surgery patients.[3] In some cases, more prolonged depressions occur, lasting weeks, months, and even years. Patients need to be better informed about what to expect during recovery, and better prepared to deal with post-operative distress.

Immediately After Surgery

Beginning immediately after surgery and continuing for about three months for some operations, the *early recovery stage* is the time when bruising and swelling are still largely in evidence. Immediately upon regaining consciousness after surgery, physical pain is often most acute, and this can precipitate remorse, fear, or anger.

> *Jackie.* The room was dark, and I heard someone say "Jackie?" I felt like I'd been run over by a train. I wasn't able to move by myself, even two or three steps to a wheelchair. I felt so frail and vulnerable! I touched my chest. It felt like someone had shoved two shoe boxes inside it. When Tony had dropped me off earlier in the morning before my breast surgery, I said I would call him after surgery and would walk the half block to the parking garage to meet him. Fat chance! I couldn't even remember our number, let alone dial the phone. Someone must have called, because he came and got me. The ride home was just miserable. With every bump in the road I thought that death sounded somehow very

inviting. I didn't think I could keep myself together for the 45-minute drive home. I thought, how could I have done this to myself?

That first week after breast surgery, Jackie was fatigued and nauseated, common problems after any surgery. She couldn't eat or sleep well. Breathing was difficult, and she complained that she itched all over. After she came down with a fever, Jackie had to be put on antibiotics to combat an infection secondary to the surgery. As if this weren't enough, she developed an allergy to the surgical tape used to keep her sutures protected. "I was told I would have lots of pain, and I expected lots of pain, but there was even more pain than I imagined there would be," reported Jackie.

Pain was not the primary issue for Paulette. She had a panic attack shortly after regaining consciousness:

Paulette. I had to travel to another town for my surgery, so I arranged to stay with a friend and her husband afterwards. He is an eye doctor. My husband took me from the surgeon's office, where the nose surgery was done, to my friend's home. Initially, I was very sleepy and didn't feel much of anything. About an hour after arriving, I started to become more aware that the inside of my nose was packed with gauze and the outside was splinted and taped. With all the packing, I couldn't breathe through my nose, forcing me to breathe through my mouth. The pressure from the packing frightened me. I felt like I might suffocate. My heart started to pound, and my palms became sweaty. I got dizzy, and I was hyperventilating. My husband and my friends tried to reassure me that everything would be okay. As the anxiety worsened, I started pulling at the packing inside my nose. Ordinarily this packing has to be in place for at least 12 hours to prevent bleeding. Mine had been in place only about 4 hours. I didn't care. I had to get it out. My husband called my surgeon, who alerted him to watch for signs of bleeding that would signal alarm and mean I would have to have the nose repacked. Fortunately, I didn't bleed. Only after the packing was removed did the panic and anxiety start to subside. I don't know what I would have done if I had had to have my nose repacked. It had never occurred to me to discuss with my doctor beforehand that I am prone to claustrophobia!

Early Recovery

Sometimes surgery triggers hidden concerns about dependency, especially for people who have a great need to feel in control of what happens to them. When such fears and anxieties are brought to the forefront by surgery or the stress of early recovery, they can trigger a personality "regression."

When this happens, perviously sensible adult behavior is replaced by behavior characteristic of a much younger age.

An example of such a problem is given by Dr. Marcia Goin.[4] A male patient who was also a powerful business executive had a skin graft on his foot. Following the operation he complained constantly, harassed the nurses, and was demanding and obnoxious. His surgeon dreaded the daily visits of this patient, whom he referred to as "an awful old man," and made them as perfunctory as possible—just long enough to attend the medical necessities. It appeared that the patient was frightened by needing to depend on others and was trying to relieve his fear that his caretakers would desert him by acting demanding and angry. When a nurse started to spend extra time with him, his attitude changed, and he became pleasant and appreciative. She changed his bandages frequently and spent time talking with him. This was not a medical necessity, but an emotional one. Once he was no longer frightened and hiding his fear behind a mask of anger, he could relax and reveal his more pleasant adult self.

Post-operative complications can cause considerable stress. About nine days after her face-lift surgery, Leanne heard a noticeable "click" in her head. In short order, her face swelled up, and she could hear a "gurgling" sound in her head. When her husband took one look at her, he said, "Come on, we're going back to the doctor." They arrived at the doctor's office at 6:30 A.M., but the nurses refused to call the doctor, saying he would be in at 8:30 A.M. Leanne's husband became quite angry at their refusal to contact the doctor, and eventually he found the doctor's home phone number in the directory and called him himself. The doctor came immediately, and Leanne was again give a local anesthetic so the doctor could drain the hematoma (blood clot) that had formed under the skin. "I'm going to look ugly the rest of my life," Leanne cried. "No, you're not," said the doctor, "fixing this is easier than doing the operation in the first place." He instructed her to spend the next few days in bed and do nothing until she was well along her way to healing.

The first few days of recovery can also be stressful for children getting ear surgery. Research has identified a number of post-operative complications that can occur.[5] Sixty-seven percent of children in the study needed to have their bandages reapplied on average 2.5 times. These tended to be younger children, who were very intolerant of the pain and who pulled at their bandages. More than half complained of pain in the first 48 hours as well as itching from the bandages. Slightly less than half experienced vomiting in the first 48 hours, and a third had the bandage come off during the night. Post-operative complications were particularly stressful for the child who was too young or unmotivated to be a willing participant. Evidence suggests that children can suffer long-term emotional consequences from invasive and painful medical procedures.[6]

Sometimes psychological distress is not apparent until days or weeks after surgery. Physical discomfort can continue for many weeks and sometimes months or even years, depending on the operation. Lauren, a 35-year-old bank teller, described her experience after having a liposuction procedure done on her thighs and buttocks:

> *Lauren.* I had always been ashamed of my fat ass and thunder thighs, and I was anxious to have liposuction, even though it would cost me $4,000. I'd done a lot of reading about it, and I thought I knew what to expect. The operation took about two hours, and I had a local anesthetic. The doctor took out two liters (about four pounds) of fat. After the anesthesia wore off, the pain really set in. I was bruised from my waist to my ankles. For weeks, I couldn't sit, and I could only lie on my stomach. The doctor had me wear a girdle-like bandage for more than a month to help the bruising and swelling go down. Finally, after six weeks, he took off the bandages. My skin looked like corrugated cardboard, and the size of my rear end and thighs didn't look any different to me. The doctor assured me it would take awhile to see the results. For months I was tender, sore, and exhausted, and I couldn't move around like I used to. I got so depressed, I started to binge eat. Within a few weeks I had gained ten pounds. They say that fat cells can't come back, once they are removed. That may be, but the remaining ones continued to store up the excess calories I started consuming. Months later, I had gained 40 pounds. I looked worse than before the surgery, and I was angry and depressed.

Significant post-operative emotional disturbances occur in 30 to 60 percent of all cosmetic surgery patients."[7] These tend to arise in the early recovery period, when pain and disfigurement from swelling and bruising have not yet abated. Such emotional disturbances tend to be depressive in nature, but can include anxiety, grief, remorse, anger, and even psychotic-like symptoms, such as delusions that certain body parts are not real. The downward swing in emotions is influenced by many factors. Disappointment or concern about seeing oneself bruised and swollen may be one. Experiencing pain, numbness, discomfort, and sensory changes is another. The negative reactions of others, or unmet expectations and dissatisfaction with the results of the operation, can contribute to post-operative psychological difficulties. Integrating a significant change of appearance into the mental image of the body can prove difficult. Finally, the anesthesia, pain, and confinement that are associated with most surgery are natural enemies of physical stamina and strength. Even a brief period of inactivity contributes to a depletion of physical functioning, including fatigue, decreased muscle strength, and deteriorating cardiovascular functioning.

With cosmetic surgery, normal functioning can be impaired, either temporarily or permanently. Patients having face-lifts occasionally experience injury to the motor nerves that can cause changes in a patient's smile and lip movement, and even contribute to some slurring of the speech. Fortunately, most patients with such injuries have a spontaneous return of normal function after several months or a year. In other cases, there may be hair loss, dislocation of the earlobes, or discoloration of the skin. Scarring is inevitable. Breast surgery can result in temporary or (rarely) permanent loss of sensation around the nipple. Nose reshaping produces numbness that endures for months. All of these factors can cause emotional distress, especially if the patient is unprepared for them.

Post-Operative Depression

Depression is not a single entity, but rather a group of disorders that range in intensity from mild feelings of "having the blues" or "feeling down" to severe, clinical depression. More severe depression is characterized by feelings of sadness or irritability that don't go away, loss of interest or pleasure in activities that used to provide enjoyment (such as hobbies or sex), a change in weight or appetite, difficulty sleeping, fatigue, inability to concentrate, or feelings of guilt, helplessness, or low self-esteem. In some cases, there are even thoughts about life not being worthwhile or about death or suicide.

Similar to patients who undergo other types of major surgery, patients who have significant cosmetic surgery are prone to depression.[8] Usually such depressive episodes are mild and short in duration. In a 1980 study of 50 face-lift patients, 54 percent had some indications of depression.[9] Mild depressive signs were found in 24 percent of patients, and 30 percent developed more intense and persistent symptoms. These symptoms emerged either immediately after the operation or within two to three weeks.

The study identified four types of patients who were most likely to suffer emotional difficulties in early recovery period. *Actives* were those who were active people and more likely to suffer transient depressions. *Belateds* were those for whom issues or stressful situations surfaced belatedly. *Controllers* preferred to be in control of their lives and were likely to succumb to longer and more serious depressions. *Dependents* tended to reject control in favor of being dependent on others. In many cases, those who developed depression after surgery had some level of pre-existing but undetected depression prior to surgery.

Actives

Actives become depressed or anxious within the first five post-operative days, but their symptoms usually disappear within the first week or two. Often such symptoms are triggered by of the physical constraints of the immediate post-operative period. Active patients are typically people who have to be doing something most of the time, and having to stay at home makes them feel like climbing the walls.

Belateds

Belateds experience temporary episodes of depression that emerge during the second or third post-operative weeks and are usually related to some new life stress, such as having a spouse suddenly become nonsupportive or actively critical, or having to respond to some unexpected crisis or situational stress. In some cases, pre-existing issues become more conscious after surgery and lead to action not consciously anticipated before, such as deciding to separate or divorce.

Controllers

Controllers usually develop depression within the first five days after surgery, and symptoms can continue for several weeks or months. Controllers are independent, self-reliant people who need to be in control of their own lives. They don't ask for support from those around them. Prior to surgery, they appear to have adequate self-esteem, and their expectation is that surgery will slow or stop the aging process. Controllers are concerned about aging, and obtaining cosmetic surgery gives them the illusion of being able to control aging. Often such patients have pre-existing though not readily apparent depression. In the post-operative period, they feel out of control of their physical experience, which deepens their depression. Their symptoms are less likely to diminish and may develop into long-lasting depressions.

Dependents

Dependents become depressed during the second or third week after surgery and remain so for several weeks or, in some cases, months. Dependents tend to be passive, and wish and need to be cared for by others. They do not want to be in control of their own lives and are less concerned about the aging process than are controllers. Like controllers, they often have pre-existing depression. They are often complaining and socially introverted, and rate the outcome of their operations less positively than other patients. Dependents seek relationships that provide strong emotional support. Recovery, for them, is a comforting, contented time, when they feel nurtured by the attention they get from those around them. However, as their recuperation progresses, this support evaporates, and they resort to their usual complaining pattern. Dawning disappointment in the results of the operation, coupled with a decrease in the emotional support from others, can precipitate the emergence of previously dormant depression.

Reactions to Breast Surgery

A large number of patients who obtain breast surgery succumb to depression. Similar to face-lift patients, these patients are often depressed before the operation as well. One study found that some degree of depression was diagnosed in 60 percent of those seeking breast augmentation.[10] Depression after breast surgery usually emerges some time between the third and the seventh days. The patterns identified for face-lift patients also occur in breast surgery patients.

For a woman, breasts are the most emotionally significant part of her body. Not only are they a highly visible sign of her femininity, they symbolize her uniquely female role as mother and nurturer. Her breasts also represent her sexuality and are a source of sensual and erotic pleasure. When the shape of the breasts is changed by the process of aging or breast-feeding, feminine pride can be grievously damaged. When a breast must be removed because of disease, it can be devastating to the patient. Even when the lost breast can be reconstructed, the woman will face psychological as well as physical scars.

The usual psychological effects of mastectomy include the panic imposed by a life-threatening disease, depression lasting for months or years, lowered self-esteem, and a diminished sense of femininity and womanliness.[11] After a mastectomy, many women experience a period of mourning.[12] The loss of their breasts can be devastating. They worry about what husbands, lovers, or people in general will think of them. The primary emotional reaction is not fear of death, but fear that femininity is endangered.[13]

The degree to which such an emotional reaction occurs for any given woman depends, of course, on her conscious attitude about her breasts, their actual appearance, and on her stage of life. Pre-existing attitudes can range from pride to indifference to revulsion and shame. Asymmetrical breasts, excessively large or small breasts, or other appearance deficits will affect attitude. Some post-menopausal women who have fulfilled their goals of marriage and motherhood reportedly have an easier time adjusting to mastectomy.[14] Others, who believe "it shouldn't matter" but for whom it does matter, have a much harder time grieving and accepting the loss.[15] Even when the breasts are a source of embarrassment and surgery is sincerely desired, breast surgery can bring mixed blessings.

Extremely large breasts, a medical condition technically termed *gigantomastia* (literally, giant breasts), can produce considerable self-consciousness because of the attention it draws. It can make psychological adjustment especially difficult for adolescents. For example, Soleil Moon Frye played the title role on the NBC sitcom *Punky Brewster* for four years, until she was 12 years old. By the time she was 15, and only five feet one, she had developed a size 38-DD bust, and boys were taunting, "Hey, Punky Boobster." A breast reduction operation helped avoid such attention and restored her self-confidence.[16]

Even though breast reduction is sought both to enhance appearance and to eliminate the back pain and other physical discomforts that giant breasts can produce, these improvements do not eliminate the potential for psychological disturbance. As with mastectomy, cuts, scars, bruises, and loss of sensitivity are inevitable concomitants of surgery. Furthermore, because a psychologically central part of the woman's body is being altered, the risk of emotional complications is high.

The most frequent initial reaction to breast reduction is euphoria, which gradually evolves into a generalized sense of well-being and heightened self-confidence and self-esteem. Sometimes those who were depressed prior to the operation (especially if depression was related to appearance) experience a lifting of the depression. Nevertheless, disturbing feelings also tend to emerge. According to one study, these can include grief for loss of a part of the body, temporary (usually) sexual and identity disturbances, and some-times body image disturbances.[17]

Because breasts are so visible and symbolic, reactions to loss or altera-tion can be severe. According to Goin and Goin, one breast reduction patient was depressed for two weeks after the operation and made the comment, "It seems weird; I've been big for so long."[18] Another woman reported a sense of loss and accompanying grief that lasted for nearly two months. She would find herself staring at big-breasted women and longing to be restored to her original size. Then she would remember that she had been miserable when she was that size, and she would "come to her senses." Still, the sense of loss continued to return.

Following breast reduction, one woman became panicked and shocked during her first sexual encounter after surgery. Her partner caressed her breasts, and she felt only pressure and no erotic sensation. Although she had been warned to expect decreased breast and nipple sensation, she underesti-mated the effect this would have on her. Yet another woman, who worried beforehand that the operation would make her breasts too small, developed a delusion that her breasts were completely gone. On the one hand she knew that her breasts were there, she could look down and see them, but subjec-tively she experienced them as gone. She was able to get through a difficult eight month adjustment period by reminding herself that she wasn't "crazy" but having a psychological reaction that would pass.

Goin and Goin also describe a patient who had an anxiety attack two weeks after her breast reduction operation. She was leaving her house on her way to the doctor's office when she suddenly experienced a strong and dis-turbing sense of having forgotten something. Despite checking and confirm-ing that she had her purse, keys, and other essentials, she still felt extremely anxious. All at once, she knew that what was missing was part of her breasts. "Something that was supposed to be there was missing," she reported. This sense of something lost or left behind continued for five weeks.

Yet another of the Goins' patients developed an uncomfortable sense of vulnerability. This was a woman who had always felt emotionally vulnerable around her mother and strangers. Her large breasts had served as a sort of "buffer" to keep others at both a physical and an emotional distance. When this patient's mother visited after the surgery, the patient became panicky and insisted that her husband stay between her mother and herself. She felt, she said, "like a turtle without its shell."

Similarly, patients who have undergone breast augmentation, can develop tearfulness lasting a few minutes to a few days when the dressings are removed, even though they insist they are happy with the results. Presumably this is a sudden discharge of emotion set off by the newly revealed alteration in body contour, rather than a truly adverse psychological reaction. Nevertheless, such tearfulness can be embarrassing and distressing to patients (as well as their doctors), because there is no apparent reason for it.

It is not uncommon for breast surgery patients to have dreams or frightening fantasies about their breasts after surgery. Jackie reported that for nearly a year after her breast lift and augmentation, she would awaken from a dream in which her breasts had shriveled up and become distorted and ugly. Following breast surgery, it is common for patients to dream that their nipples fall off or to experience their breasts as "pasted on," not their own, or foreign.

After breast surgery, patients tend to touch their breasts a great deal, often in the dark. This is not a form of sexual or masturbatory activity but an exploration of their newly altered body contour. Seeing and feeling their breasts is the way they come to accept the change as truly part of themselves. Unlike those who have had other types of cosmetic surgery operations, patients who have had breast augmentation are often quite pleased to show their breasts to others.

Reactions to Nose Reshaping

Pat was a 34-year-old unmarried, plain-looking nurse who had always been shy and jealous of her younger, married, and more outgoing sister. In the family she was seen as troubled, sad, lonely, and emotionally disappointed. She hated her nose, which she felt was mainly responsible for her difficulties. After having a rhinoplasty, she underwent a period of dejected seclusion till her "black eyes" went away. She was embarrassed by the visible evidence of her effort to change her appearance. Not only did the nose reshaping not change her social or emotional situation, her family devalued her actions by remarking, "It doesn't really look like you."

Roger was a 36-year-old executive who told the surgeon that he wanted a complete makeover of his nose. In fact, it was a heavy, ill-defined nose that was deviated and slightly asymmetric. He wanted his nose to be straight and narrow with a refined "chiseled" tip. At first Roger was happy with the results, until major reversals occurred in his business. He began to question his decision to have such a refined tip, and blamed his business difficulties on his significantly changed appearance.

The nose is the most prominent feature of the face, and its size and shape are important to appearance. Although the nose does most of its growing during puberty, it continues to enlarge throughout life, though very slowly. Most people don't realize that the nose ages along with the rest of the face. Gradually the base widens, the tip begins to droop, and a prominent hump can appear. In some cases, the skin thickens and discolors, mistakenly giving an alcoholic appearance.

Although most patients are happy with the results of a rhinoplasty, sometimes severe emotional difficulties arise after a nose reshaping operation. In one study, nine female rhinoplasty patients experienced adverse psychological reactions that developed from altered perceptions while under local anesthesia. Being drugged but retaining some level of consciousness and being physically restrained and sensorially deprived contributed to delusions. Often the delusion was triggered by overhearing conversation and misinterpreting ambiguous comments made during the operation. Some patients reported believing that their operation was performed by an "assistant learning on them" and that their own surgeon didn't do the operation. Six of the nine patients said that the surgeon and his assistant argued over the proper technique to use during the operation. All of the nine experienced a panic-like state while under local anesthesia, and said they felt assaulted. Following the operation they made numerous physical complaints, requested additional surgery for revision of "mistakes" they felt had occurred, and publicly ridiculed their surgeons. In all nine cases, there was a gradual deterioration in their relationships with their surgeons, and one even threatened a law suit.

Literature, myth, and folklore are replete with stories of the emotional, psychological, and symbolic significance of the nose. Gogol's famous short story, *The Nose*, is about a petty government official who awakens to discover his nose has inexplicably vanished. Later he finds it on the face of a lofty superior. He becomes preoccupied with his image and tries repeatedly to get back his nose. The story illustrates how the nose symbolizes his masculinity, his worldly ambitions, his prospects for marriage, and his very identity as a person. In Edmond Rostand's play, Cyrano de Bergerac is the long-nosed tragic hero who, ashamed to face the woman he loves, suffered the pain and sorrow of unrequited love. The ancient Romans, and even some modern day Italians, believed that the size of the nose was an indicator of the size of the penis. Historically, adultery has been punished by amputation of the nose. In fact, the first nose surgery originated thousands of years ago in India to correct the results of such punishment.

Most people who have their noses reshaped are ultimately happy with the results, even though they must endure initial pain, discomfort, and embarrassment. Paulette described her first few weeks and her first venture out in public after surgery:

> *Paulette.* One of the worst things was that I couldn't wash my hair for a week. For weeks, I had to sleep propped up in a sitting position, and keep head movements to a minimum, no heavy work or looking down. It took more than a month to get my physical strength back. After four weeks, I went out to run errands and go to the supermarket. I still had a strip over the bridge of my nose, but I didn't care if people knew I had a nose job. I was very ex-

cited and eager to see my nose. I was told it takes six months to a year before my nose would take its final shape. After six weeks I got my first look. It was gorgeous! It was totally numb, and this didn't go away for almost a year, so it didn't feel like a part of my body, but it looked great. For the first time, I enjoyed making up my eyes because my nose was finally in proportion to the rest of my face.

Psychological Distress and Early Recovery

Susan Shore, Ph.D., a psychologist who investigated the recovery experiences of cosmetic surgery patients, argues that post-operative trauma and depression are much higher than have been formerly reported.[19] Her research indicates that patients are not adequately prepared for the amount of pain that can occur, the shock of seeing themselves disfigured (even if temporarily) because of bruising and swelling, or the physical toll of fatigue and loss of stamina that major surgery exacts on the body. These elements combine with surprise, confusion, and uncertainty to create significant emotional distress, both initially and in the weeks and months following surgery.

Plastic surgeons undertake their profession at least in part because they want to help others and to obtain the approval and gratitude of their patients. Surgeons are naturally distressed when a patient has any kind of difficulty after surgery, including difficult emotional reactions. It can be easier to view the patient's problem by covertly blaming the patient or the patient's family—her expectations were unrealistic, she did it for the wrong reasons, she had pre-existing depression, the family is unsupportive, marital problems already existed. It is certainly true that psychological difficulties after cosmetic surgery can be caused or exacerbated by these factors and others, including the impact of the change on a patient's mental image of her- or himself. Nevertheless, both surgeons and patients must be prepared to cope with the psychological difficulties that can occur after surgery, regardless of the causes.

Pre-Existing Depression

Doctors argue that cosmetic surgery patients who develop depression after surgery were most likely depressed beforehand. If such depression was not clearly evident prior to surgery, then it must have been "masked." That is, the patient, either consciously or subconsciously, kept it hidden from the surgeon. This explanation conveniently shifts the major responsibility for the depression to the patient.

Certainly patients with pre-existing depression are likely to be a greater risk for post-operative depression. In fact, those seeking cosmetic surgery are likely to have relatively high levels of pre-existing depression, mainly because these potential patients are primarily older women. Women are twice as likely as men to develop depression.[20] They experience higher rates of physical and sexual abuse (predictors of later depression) and their role conditioning encourages patterns of negative thinking and passivity.[21] For some women, depression is related to hormonal changes such as premenstrual syndrome, childbirth, and menopause. In addition, women seeking cosmetic surgery are generally at the middle stage of life, when the risk of depression generated by the inevitable losses and disappointments in life naturally increases.

According to a 1981 study, at any given time the prevalence of depressive symptoms in the general population ranges between 9 and 20 percent, depending on the criteria used to define depression and how the diagnosis is made.[22] With more liberal criteria and when people self-report their symptoms, the prevalence reaches 40 percent.[23] Therefore, every middle-aged woman seeking cosmetic surgery should be assumed to be at risk for depression, and both patient and surgeon need to be prepared to deal with this potential problem.

Recognizing Symptoms of Psychological Distress

Depression is the "common cold" of emotional difficulties. Nearly half of all men and three-quarters of women are at risk for developing some symptoms of depression at any given time. Although it is the most prevalent mental health problem, it is by no means a mild complaint.[24] A clinical or "major" depression differs from the depressed or sad mood that normally accompanies life's losses or disappointments. One out of ten men and one out of four women will experience a clinical depression at least once during their lifetimes. Of those who succumb to major depression, 50 percent will relapse within two years.[25] In some cases clinical depression can be fatal; it is responsible for most suicide deaths. Depression also significantly impacts relationships and family life, as well as workplace functioning. In addition, depression adversely affects the immune system and the body's capacity to combat physical disorders.[26]

The symptoms of clinical depression vary enormously from one person to another, but if at least five of the symptoms listed under *Symptoms of Major Depression* are present during the same two-week period and represent a change from previous experience, it is highly likely that a major depression is present.

Seeking Help

Most depressions, especially those that are caused by upsetting events, have a natural course and gradually improve over time, usually within six months. When depression doesn't start to improve in a few months, or when there are symptoms of a major depression, especially if accompanied by thoughts of death or suicide, the help of a mental health professional should be sought. Usually this is either a psychiatrist or a psychologist. Although the first stop is sometimes the family doctor, primary care physicians often fail to recognize depression in their patients.[27]

The two main approaches to treatment for depression are medication and psychotherapy. Medication is generally indicated for the more severe depressions. New anti-depressant medications such as Prozac have fewer side effects than older tricyclics, though no one anti-depressant medication is more clearly effective than another, and no single medication results in remission for all patients. The overall efficacy of medication for relieving symptoms of depression is about 58 percent.[28] Patients generally start to experience symptom relief within six weeks of beginning medication, but even if symptoms improve, many patients may still have problems with daily functioning. Pills alone rarely cure depression entirely. When difficulties in coping with life continue to persist, psychotherapy may be beneficial.

Symptoms of Major Depression

1. Feeling depressed most of the day, nearly every day. (Children and adolescents can appear irritable.)

2. Not being interested, or taking less pleasure in all or almost all activities that previously gave satisfaction.

3. Having lost more than 5 percent of body weight in a month when not dieting, or having gained weight, especially associated with carbohydrate craving.

4. Experiencing a decrease or increase in appetite nearly every day, especially in the absence of ability to enjoy food.

5. Having difficulty falling asleep or staying asleep, or sleeping too much.

6. Feeling tense, anxious, or unable to sit still, or feeling slow and unable to move.

7. Feeling fatigued or having a loss of energy every day.

8. Feeling worthless or very guilty (not about being sick) nearly every day, or engaging in excessive self-pity or self-blame.

9. Having thoughts of death (not just fear of dying), or thinking about suicide.

10. Crying frequently or feeling emotionally flat or dead.

11. Having difficulty concentrating, or having intrusive thoughts or worries, especially worries about health.

12. Feeling irritable or quick to anger.

Psychotherapy can take several different forms, two of which are cognitive therapy and interpersonal therapy. Cognitive therapy focuses on changing the negative thoughts and interpretations of events that depressed people usually engage in that perpetuate depression. Interpersonal therapy deals with problems of grief, conflicts among family and friends, life transitions, and interpersonal deficits. In this approach, it is assumed that symptoms of current emotional problems result from the need to survive in a social environment determined partly by childhood experience and partly by present-day relationships. For mild to moderate depressions, these and other brief forms of psychotherapy have an efficacy rate of approximately 50 percent. Persons with more severe or chronic depression, or who do not get complete relief from either medication or psychotherapy alone, may be better served with a combination of medication and psychotherapy.

A tantalizing question is, can depression be prevented? There is reason to think that prior experience with the disorder may increase subsequent risk. A person who has had a single episode of major depression has a 50 percent risk of it recurring. A person who has had two or more such episodes has between a 70 and 90 percent risk of recurrence. Negative life events, which usually trigger at least the first episode of major depression, may sensitize key neural structures and pave the way for later depression, with or without the involvement of new stressors.

To prevent depression, those at risk first need to be identified and provided with appropriate assistance. Prospective cosmetic surgery patients comprise one group that is clearly at risk. To reduce their risk of post-operative emotional distress, these patients need to be as fully informed about all aspects of the recovery process and realistically prepared for the pain, discomfort, depression, and second thoughts that are likely to accompany recuperation from this type of major surgery.

Summary

Most patients underestimate the amount of pain and physical trauma involved in cosmetic surgery. They are also unprepared for the emotional consequences, especially the depression (usually short-term) that may ensue. When depression doesn't pass in a reasonable time, it may be necessary to seek professional help.

I was glad to get home to my own bed. A friend agreed to stay with me during the first few days to change the compresses on my eyes and tend to my needs in general. This was a lifesaver, because I was too weak to do much more than stay in bed. Although the pain had begun to abate, I still had to take pain medication regularly. The constriction under my chin and the discomfort over the top of my head continued unrelentingly.

The day after I got home, I finally got to take a shower and wash my hair. It was caked with dried blood and stuck together in places. Parts of my scalp were tender to touch. Other parts were numb. As I stepped into the shower I felt slightly dizzy. I let the warm water gently wash over my head and down my back. Gingerly I patted shampoo into my hair. I was afraid to rub too vigorously. My scalp felt like a foreign object, something that was not mine exactly, but that I was handling at a distance. I could feel the swelling and the heavy metal staples that pulled together the two folds of skin where the incision had been made for my forehead lift.

After patting myself dry, I decided to take my first look. The face I saw in the mirror was a shock. My eyes were now open, though still significantly swollen. Purple-red bruises covered the entire eye socket and underneath. Black stitches were visible along the inside crease of my lids, extending to the corners of my eyes. Gone were the familiar furrows between my eyebrows and the lines in my forehead. Gone too was my ability to move any part of my forehead or my eyebrows. Lines of black stitches began at the base of each ear and proceeded in front to the top of each ear, extending for about an inch toward my eyebrows. These lines marked where the skin and underlying tissues had been pulled up and back to eliminate sagging cheeks. As a result, my mouth was pulled into a tight horizontal line. When I talked my mouth didn't work quite right, and I slurred some of my words. The skin of my jaw where it met my ears was blotchy red. Although I couldn't see it, a suture line also extended behind each ear and into my hairline. My whole face was puffy and swollen, giving it a round shape. I couldn't help thinking, as I saw my reflection, that it looked a lot like *Mad Magazine's* Alfred E. Newman. All I needed were freckles!

As I stood there seeing my image for the first time, I had little comprehension of the long recovery process ahead of me. I did not know then that the sensation of a strap cinched tightly under my chin and over the top of my head would continue for years. I did not yet know that my ear lobes had been sutured to the surrounding skin so that less lobe was available, and that I would always have trouble wearing earrings. I was not yet aware that the incisions in front of and behind my ears would develop large, itchy, sensitive scars that interfered with wearing glasses and that required injections, massage, and many months to abate. I did not know that I would temporarily lose hair around my hairline and that the skin of my jaw would be permanently discolored. What I saw was disturbing. It didn't look like me, and it didn't feel like me. Something was lost. A sense of sadness welled up. I wasn't yet able to appreciate the potential—to realize that the frown lines, the sleepy look, the sagging cheeks and neck were gone. At this moment, there was only uncertainty and physical discomfort.

8

Mirror, Mirror . . .
Who Is That?

When I looked in the mirror, the face reflected there not only didn't look like me, it didn't *feel* like me. My forehead and eyebrows felt stiff, and my face felt like a mask. My immobilized muscles could no longer provide others with the nonverbal cues humans use to help communicate—a raise of the eyebrow, a furrowing of the brow, a hint of a smile. Anger, sadness, joy didn't play across my frozen forehead. My smile was now asymmetrical and constricted. What's more, sensing my own feelings was difficult. I had learned in my training that feelings, emotions, and moods are partly the result of noticing certain experiences in the body, such as clenched fists, a hot face, bulging veins, a slumped posture, a silly grin, a pounding heart, or a queasy stomach. Such *proprioceptive feedback* (information originating in muscles, tendons, and other internal tissues) is interpreted by the mind as emotion. I had not realized before the extent to which smiling, frowning, and flexing other muscles in the face told *me* what emotions I was feeling.

In addition to the changes in my experience of my emotional self, surgery brought disturbing sensory and tactile changes. Numbness extended from just in front of my ear, down the side of my cheek to the cheekbone, and over to my chin, as if someone had injected me with novocaine. At night, I couldn't feel the pillow under my head. Putting on makeup was like touching someone else's face. The familiar sensation of my husband touching my face had changed to the unfamiliar. The skin on my neck had become unusually sensitive, and high collars and turtlenecks caused such irritation that I had to avoid wearing them.

It didn't matter that everyone said I looked terrific—and ten years younger. I didn't look like myself, and I didn't feel like myself. I had lost touch with who I thought I was, and it was terrifying.

The Concept of Body Image

Body image is the major key to understanding motivation for cosmetic surgery and recovery. The plastic surgeon/psychiatrist team of John and Marcia Goin define *body image* as the mental representation or perception a person has of his or her body at any given moment in time.[1] Simplistically, body image is the picture of the body as seen through the mind's eye. It is made up of perceptions, thoughts, attitudes, emotions, and concepts about the body. The physical experience of posture, size, weight, location in space, and tactile and inner sensations contribute to this image. Body image encompasses the emotional significance of the body as a whole, as well as its various parts. These parts are the surface of the body and its contours and appendages, such as the nose, ears, arms, or legs.

Body image is not the same as self-image, self-esteem, or self-concept, although body image is part of self-concept. The term "self" has been used in a variety of ways by philosophers, psychologists, and writers. Freud used self to indicate a set of mental processes operating to satisfy inner drives.[2] For Eric Erikson, self referred to individual identity and continuity of personal character.[3] Erich Fromm[4] and Abraham Maslow[5] used self to refer to the "inner nature" or "essential nature." Carl Rogers[6] conceived of the self as the meaning-making system of the personality, which provides for psychological adaptation and growth. Others have used self to refer to the experience and content of self-awareness.[7] Still others argue that self is the subjective experience of being an active agent that effects change.[8]

In line with this last concept, self refers to the subjective experience of being in the world, as known through the senses and through thinking, perceiving, remembering, reasoning, and attending. The self is not simply a repository of knowledge and evaluation of one's being. Such a fund of knowledge is termed "self-concept." Body image is one aspect of self-concept. "Self-image" is an individual's picture of himself or his personality. "Self-esteem" is the product of the person's comparison of his or her notion of the ideal self and the actual self as perceived by that person—including the body image.

How Body Image Develops

Influenced by interpersonal, environmental, and temporal factors, body image begins to emerge in infancy and continues to develop and change throughout the life cycle. Each person organizes and constructs his or her body image through the integration of many perceptions and experiences over a lifetime. Individual personality factors and outside influences such as the reactions of others affect body image.

Infants begin to experience their bodies through exploration, play, touch, and interaction with caregivers, laying the foundation for body image. In the beginning, the infant is unable to tell where he begins and ends. Gradually he begins to distinguish himself from the outside world. At first only certain parts are perceived: the mouth is separate from mom's breast, the foot is different from a rattle. As the infant discovers the boundaries of his body, the body image begins to coalesce. Around six months of age, the infant is fully aware of his separateness, and he becomes exceedingly anxious when a caregiver leaves his presence. This early anxiety about abandonment remains dormant in our experience, but can reawaken under certain circumstances, such as the loss of a loved one or the loss of a body part.

Babies and children who are held and cuddled and provided with praise and acceptance have a good start toward a positive body image. Those who lack positive physical contact or are subjected to criticism, derision, or rejection may fail to develop the ability to view their body realistically. A fascination with the appearance of others begins at about six months of life and is more pronounced and more actively sought by babies for whom mothering has been inadequate, when the mother is emotionally unavailable to the child or out of step with the infant's needs. Such infants grow up with an intense longing for acceptance and and may value appearance as a means of gaining approval from others.

Somewhere between two and four years of age, the sense of "being a boy" or "being a girl" develops, and the socialization of boys and girls begins to diverge. Each learns how a "pretty girl" or a "handsome boy" looks and behaves. Boys are more roughly handled and played with than girls and are punished more, thus learning to value physical prowess and tolerate physical discomfort. Whereas little boys are rewarded for achievements, little girls are praised for looking and acting nice. While boys are allowed virtually free run or a room, girls learn to take up less space and engage in finer actions. Both soon learn society's standards of "beautiful," and how these apply differently to boys and girls. Failure to measure up, significant rejection by adults or peers, or negative messages from parents can impair body image development at an early age.

> *Phyllis.* Phyllis was the older of two daughters and the only natural-born child of her mother; her younger sister was adopted. As long as Phyllis could remember, her mother had labeled her "fragile" and "sickly," declaring her sister to be the healthy and "robust one." Despite her good grades in school, her mother worried that Phyllis wouldn't make it. At age 53, Phyllis's body image was that of a weak, sickly person who could barely get through the day. On the advice of a therapist Phyllis took up bodybuilding with

the help of a personal trainer. Under his direction and with the encouragement of her therapist, Phyllis's newly found strengths and abilities began to improve her body image. For the first time in her life Phyllis began to see herself as strong.

Although body image continues to evolve throughout life, adolescence is a particularly difficult time. Adjusting to changes in body image is a major psychological task. Surveys of young adolescents confirm high degrees of anxious body preoccupation and dissatisfaction. Generally, girls are more dissatisfied than boys. The recent epidemic rise in eating disorders, which are associated with body image dissatisfaction, and the spread of dieting behavior into grade school indicates that body image is a great source of psychological turmoil and a big stumbling block in adolescent development. Parental attitudes and reactions to a teenager's physical changes, sociocultural factors, and the teenager's personality contribute to either positive or negative changes in body image during adolescence.

Body image is complex and dynamic. Although it usually reaches a level of stability by adulthood, small fluctuations and changes can and do occur over short periods of time. Even during a single day body image can vary. For example, after strenuous exercise a person may feel thin for a while and then, a few hours later, after eating may feel bloated and fat. Over the long term, body image develops and changes as a result of what other people say about one's body, how they react to it, and how the person reacts to key events experienced in the course of life.

Frank. When Frank was seven years old his mother died. Frank and his younger brother were sent to live with their maternal grandparents. About a year later, Frank's father and new wife took custody of Frank and his brother and moved to another state. Frank's father and stepmother immediately began to criticize Frank for being too fat. They withheld food from him, ridiculed his appearance, or taunted him, calling him "fatty" and "piggy." In addition to the verbal abuse, Frank's father frequently beat him. The more unhappy and angry Frank became, the more he ate, and the more he ate, the more he came to despise himself and his body. At age 40, Frank was six feet tall and weighed 290 pounds. Still single, he ate when he felt lonely and he ate when he felt angry. At age 37 he went on a weight reducing program and lost 50 pounds, but he still felt ugly and unhappy. Eating allowed him to blot out feelings about his body, even though afterwards he felt bloated and his self-loathing was worse. He regained all the weight he had lost.

In the beginning, body image is quite flexible. Consequently, children and young people have a much easier time adapting to changes wrought through cosmetic surgery. With increasing age, the body image solidifies, and adapting to changes is more difficult. In adults, adjustment in body image appears to lag behind actual physical changes. Thus, a woman who loses a large amount of weight and reaches goal weight may still experience herself as fat, and a man who has always been thin but who gains weight later in life may still see himself as being at normal weight. Older patients seeking cosmetic surgery are reportedly less able to cope with significant changes in appearance than younger patients because the body image has become relatively fixed.[9] When surgery causes more change than can easily be assimilated by the patient's body image, a severe reaction is possible. Michael Pertschuk, M.D., of the Center for Human Appearance at the University of Pennsylvania School of Medicine reported the following case of Sara, who encountered such a problem:[10]

> *Sara.* Sara, a 32-year-old single business woman, underwent surgery to correct a temporal mandibular joint (TMJ) problem, which involved significantly altering the position of her jaw. Her profile was improved by the surgery, and her face was shortened. Cosmetically, the results were dramatic but largely unanticipated by the patient. During the two weeks following surgery, Sara developed anxiety attacks requiring psychiatric intervention. In therapy she described being "unnerved" by the difference in her reflection in the mirror. Even though she liked what she saw, it did not look like her. She was also unsettled by the reactions of friends who at first failed to recognize her. Eventually her psychiatric symptoms abated as she increasingly came to accept her new face as her own.

Reportedly, men have more difficulty adapting to changes induced by cosmetic surgery than women. This may be because men do not have a tradition of altering their appearance with cosmetics, hair color and style, and clothes, at least not to the extent women do. Men are less critical of their appearance than women are, and this may contribute to their having a more fixed body image. Far fewer men than women seek cosmetic surgery, and it may be that those who do are more prone to becoming disturbed by the effects of cosmetic surgery.

Body Boundaries

Body image defines the boundaries of the body, that is, where the body begins and ends in space. The sense of body boundaries makes it possible to move about a room without bumping into furniture or other people. Body image and its sense of boundaries helps a person scratch the exact spot that itches.

Not only do people know where their bodies begin and end, they also have some notion of the space around them they consider their own. This "comfort zone" of personal space differs from person to person, from situation to situation, and from culture to culture. Latin Americans have a smaller comfort zone than North Americans. People in a crowded subway tolerate closer proximity to others than when in a park. People of the same age, gender, and social class, are allowed to be closer than those who are different. When the comfort zone is invaded, or is no longer discernable, people become uncomfortable and anxious. In some cases, an interruption of body boundaries can lead to disintegration of the mental picture of the body and to psychic instability.

Sudden alterations or transformations of the body are the theme of many stories and myths. From *The Portrait of Dorian Gray* to *Pinocchio* and *The Little Mermaid*, both adult and children's literature show an awareness of, and concern for, body image. The breach of body boundaries in cosmetic surgery touches a fear that has lurked in the human collective unconscious since the beginning of time. Cosmetic surgery can be experienced as an invasion of body boundaries and can cause at least a temporary destabilization of body image for some people.

Distortion and Disturbance of Body Image

Virtually everyone experiences some parts of their bodies as bigger, smaller, flatter, rounder, longer, shorter, or more or less desirable than is actually the case by objective standards. A body image *distortion* is a discrepancy between what might be objectively true and what is subjectively experienced. This distortion is quite common. People who lose substantial weight may still think of themselves as fat, despite now being thinner. In spite of wrinkles, bags, and sags many older people say they still think of themselves as much younger, say 25 or 35. Usually there is a time lag between the occurrence of changes in the body and revision of the body image to reflect these changes.

Nearly everyone has some degree of body image distortion because there is rarely a one-to-one correspondence between objective and subjective reality. Distortions are generated by beliefs and attitudes that are culturally learned and transmitted. Body image distortion can also follow routine plastic surgery, though such a problem is usually temporary, lasting a few weeks or months. Nevertheless, such body image distortions can cause much anxiety and even the fear of "going crazy." When such distortions reach delusional proportions, a body image *disturbance* can be said to exist.

A body image disturbance involves an extremely negative reaction or attitude toward the body, and may in some cases include an aversion to the whole body or some part of it. Unlike a body image distortion, a body image disturbance causes significant anxiety and interferes with the ability to carry out daily activities, have satisfactory relationships, make good judgements, or experience positive emotions. Disturbances of body image can be quite serious and can lead some people to seek repeated surgical procedures or drastic alterations of appearance. In rare cases, surgery itself can produce a body image disturbance. When appearance is significantly altered, a few patients may experience a psychological reaction that significantly interferes with the ability to function. A sudden change to a body part can elicit such anxiety that the patient may develop the delusion that the body part is severely damaged, diseased, or otherwise objectionable, even though no objective evidence of this exists.

Body Image and Eating Disorders

Dissatisfaction with body image is the hallmark of an eating disorder. An integral part of both anorexia nervosa and bulimia is a preoccupation with and desire to change body shape and weight. Through stringent dieting or purging, an eating-disordered person seeks to mold her body into an "acceptable" shape. Such people may also seek cosmetic surgery. They are motivated by a poor and distorted body image. Even though surgery often produces initial satisfaction and an improvement in body image the results are almost always short-lived, and dissatisfaction with body image returns, along with disordered eating behavior. An article in the *New Zealand Medical Journal* reported the experience of Ellen.[11]

> *Ellen.* Ellen's eating disorder began at the age of 17. After gaining weight with her first pregnancy, she became extremely dissatisfied with her body shape and weight. After losing weight as the result of a brief illness, she continued her weight loss trend by inducing vomiting after eating any food, even very small amounts. At age 21 she was diagnosed with anorexia nervosa with intermittent binge eating, regular vomiting, dieting, and excessive exercise. Binge eating became regular at 28, during a pregnancy and continued with no remission until she sought treatment for an eating disorder at age 40. Ellen first considered breast augmentation surgery at 36 during a period when her bulimia was severe and after a negative comment by her spouse about the size of her breasts. She became increasingly dissatisfied with her breast size over the next year, and at age 37 sought surgery. The breast enhancement did not help resolve her extremely low self-esteem or dissatisfaction with her body. Her first surgery was followed by several operative procedures to correct considerable scarring resulting from the initial surgery, which further impaired her already poor self-image. With psychotherapy she came to understand that the same body image disturbance that led to her eating disorder also instigated her motivation for cosmetic surgery.

Disturbances in Body Image from Cosmetic Surgery

Cosmetic surgery can have a significant impact on body image that requires a psychological readjustment and adaptation to a new self. Most patients experience some psychological distress following surgery, though this is usually mild and abates within weeks. During this period patients may be irritable, weepy, and emotionally up and down. Some patients are not able to make the adjustment to a difference in appearance as in the case of Connie.[12]

> *Connie.* Connie was a 26-year-old woman who had had a rhinoplasty two years earlier. Despite an objectively good result, Connie was devastated with the surgical outcome, complaining that she no longer recognized herself in the mirror. Two additional nose operations by other surgeons were unsuccessful in recapturing her original nasal appearance. Connie became psychotically depressed and was psychiatrically hospitalized. Against the medical advice of her psychiatrist, Connie continued to insist on surgery to restore her previous appearance. She wanted a widening and lengthening of the nasal tip, which was in conflict with the usual norm of attractiveness. Most patients and surgeons prefer a thinner, more sculptured nasal tip to the rounded shape Connie requested. Further investigation found that the fatter nasal tip was more consistent with Connie's internal body image. Another surgeon undertook the patient's request and "plumped out" the nasal tip. Connie was delighted with the surgical outcome, and her depression lifted. A follow-up four years later revealed that Connie had maintained her psychological improvement and had sought no additional surgery. She needed no further psychiatric treatment after having brought her actual appearance into line with her body image.

Restorative operations such as the classic face-lift seldom cause serious body image disturbances because the basic appearance is unchanged. Presumably the patient has a mental image of how she used to look years earlier, and surgery merely restores an appearance that matches this memory. With a restorative operation, friends commonly remark on how well the patient looks and attribute this to weight loss or a new hairstyle. A minor body image disturbance may occur after a face-lift, but this is often due to changes in skin sensation. If patients are not warned to expect temporary numbness of the skin on the face and neck, they may report feeling strange, uneasy, or anxious, not realizing that the boundaries between self and non-self have been blurred.

Radical face-lifts, nose reshapings, and breast reductions or augmentations, which substantially change the appearance, can be associated with more extensive body image disturbances and give rise to considerable distress. When an appearance-changing operation is done, such as the "oriental" eyelid operation (when an eyelid fold is created where none existed before), there can be disturbance. Patients may report a loss of identity: "I'm not myself anymore." The Goins indicate that body image disturbances after eyelid surgery may be more common than assumed. Also, mild, short-lived reactions in rhinoplasty patients are not uncommon while they become accustomed to their new appearance.

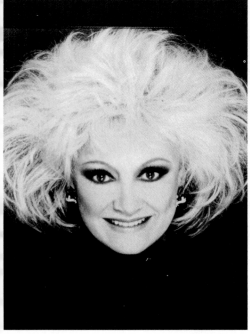

Phyllis Diller   1989

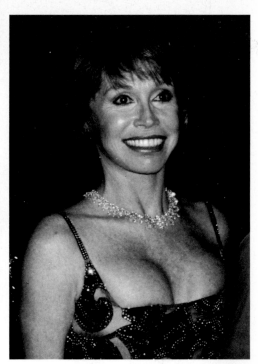

Mary Tyler Moore   1990

1968

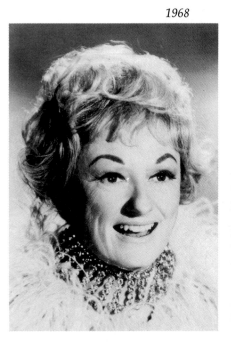

1979

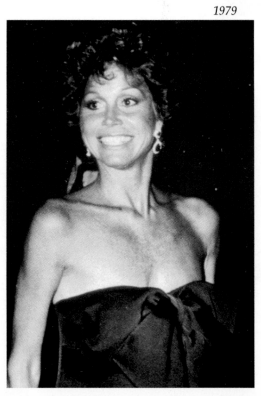

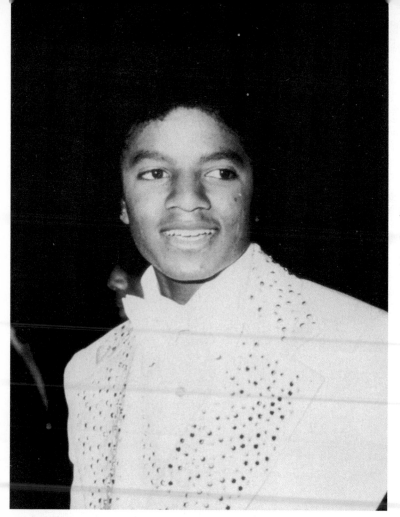

Michael Jackson

1977

1980

1981

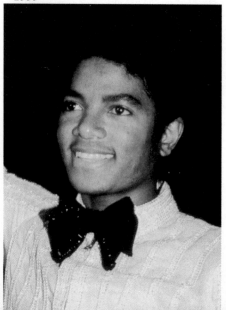

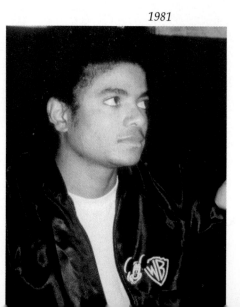

1993

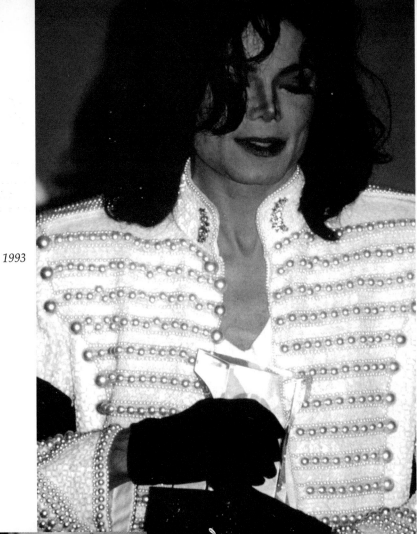

1983

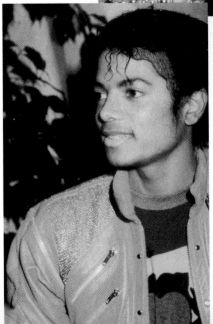

1989

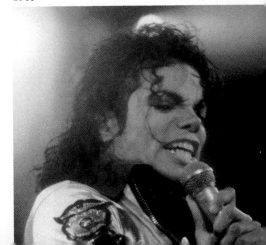

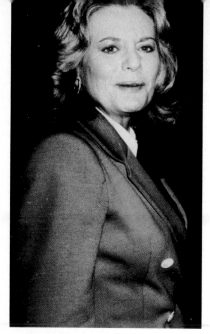

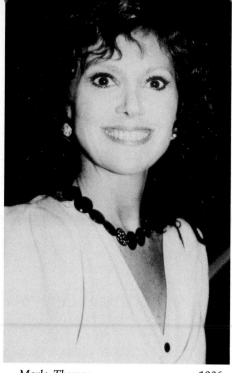

Barbara Walters   1980

1982

Marlo Thomas   1986

1985

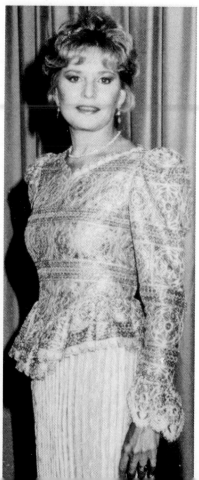

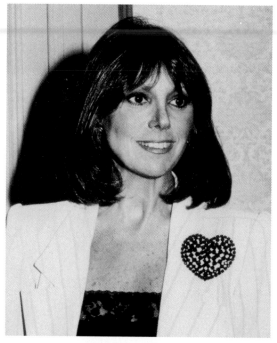

Uneasiness or anxiety about change in the body should not be confused with pleasure or displeasure with the physical results of an operation. Patients can be delighted with the surgical outcome and still suffer a relatively severe body image disturbance. Psychotic reactions are rare but can happen.

Emotional Significance of Parts of the Body

Since earlier than the time of Helen of Troy, who had "the face that launched a thousand ships," the face has been acknowledged to have special meaning in human experience. It is an important signifier of character and an immediate indicator of ethnic background. By expression and animation the face conveys emotional states. People of different cultures identify the same emotions from facial expressions. Emotions are often difficult to hide, and the face can betray the true feelings that may be denied verbally.

The eyes and nose are the focal point of the face and of appearance, and any aesthetic change to the eyes makes a big change in appearance. The eyes express both character and emotion. It is not just the eyeball but rather the associated structures, the eyelids, brows, muscle, skin, and orbital rim, that convey expression.

Surgical changes to any facial feature can result in powerful feelings that range from joy and increased self-confidence to grief for the loss of identification with a cultural heritage. The nose is particularly important as an indicator of ethnicity. How a patient feels about his or her family or ethnic group contributes to the psychological impact of cosmetic surgery on the nose. As discussed earlier, the nose has been reported to have sexual symbolism for both men and women. Some argue that for men, the nose–penis "equation" has significant potential for provoking psychological disturbance. In one case, a man presumably had unconscious conflicts about his sexual identity that became displaced onto concerns about the size and shape of his nose. After his rhinoplasty, he became paranoid and developed the delusion that his nose was slowly rotting and would eventually disappear.

John and Marcia Goin discuss the particular significance that breasts hold for women.[13] Breasts are a sign of motherliness, sexuality, and femininity. They symbolize the uniquely female role of mother. Breasts not only provide the means for feeding and nurturing the infant, they symbolize the entirety of maternal feelings and drives. Breasts are also sexual. They are a source of sensual and erotic pleasure and a way to attract and interest a potential mate. More than any other body part, breasts represent femininity.

One study compared 64 women who were to undergo or already had undergone breast augmentation with a control group of 28 women undergoing surgery other than plastic surgery.[14] The women who wanted breast augmentation were generally less certain of themselves and felt less feminine. More than 80 percent of the augmentation patients reported feeling conspicuously unfeminine with their "small" breasts and sometimes pointed out their "masculine" features, such as having broad shoulders. They also felt that women with bigger breasts were more feminine than those with smaller breasts. They tended to compare themselves to a cultural ideal of beauty rather than to other women. Ten percent of the augmentation patients thought they had "no breasts at all" despite the fact their breasts were a normal size. The body images of 90 percent of the plastic surgery patients were not realistic. In order to feel "normal," they believed their breasts had to be bigger. The investigators concluded that women who want breast augmentation are insecure in their female role, and for them feeling feminine is connected with breast size.

Breasts are often a woman's most prized possession. According to some psychoanalysts, the breast has the same psychological and emotional meaning for a woman that the penis does for a man. The loss of a breast for a woman can feel as degenderizing as castration in males.

Penis size is frequently mentioned in jokes and literature. Almost always, bigger is better. A small penis is an object of derision. In *Male Sexuality*, Bernie Zilbergeld discusses the "fantasy model of sex" that men are led to believe is reality.[15] According to the fantasy, women crave nothing so much as "a penis that might be mistaken for a telephone pole" and an "erection a mile long." Not only are these fantasyland penises larger than life, literature reports their doing strange things—throbbing, pulsating, and leaping out of a man's pants. No wonder ordinary men who fall for this fantasy—but whose penises neither look nor act like this—are sensitive about such matters. The penis is the man's badge of masculinity. It is easy for a man's fears and anxieties about other issues to be manifested as concerns about his sexuality and the size of his penis. Playing on these fears, some physicians are promoting cosmetic techniques for enlarging or lengthening the penis. Most plastic surgeons regard such operations as ill-advised.

Impact of Cosmetic Surgery on Body Image

Cosmetic surgery not only changes the visual appearance of the patient, it alters physical sensation, emotional reactions, and self-perception. A type-changing operation (one that alters, rather than merely restores a former appearance) can cause anxiety and a disturbance in body image even when the results are objectively good, because the newly altered appearance no longer matches the patient's mental picture. Usually the body image adjusts over time to the changed appearance and anxiety abates.

Changes in physical sensation, numbness, pain, sensitivity, and itching, can also significantly impact body image. One study found that 98 percent of women obtaining orthodontic surgery had some loss of sensation in the lips and chin immediately after surgery. Of these, 26 percent had a full return of sensation within 12 to 24 months, and 25 percent had a partial return of sensation within the same time period.[16] A change or loss of physical sensation blurs body boundaries and can induce considerable anxiety for those who are not forewarned. Dr. Marcia Goin described a patient who had difficulty finding the part of her breast that itched in order to scratch it.[17] The patient complained, "What used to be in one place is now in another."

Breast surgery, more than other types of operations, appears to induce body image disturbances, most of which are temporary. Having dreams and nightmares after surgery are not uncommon for those who have had breast surgery. Goin and Goin reported that one of their patients dreamed that her nipples fell off when the sutures were removed.[18] Another had the persistent feeling that her breasts were "pasted on," not her own, and liable to fall off at any moment. (Fears that nipples are sewed on and liable to fall off may be the result of the breast-reduction patient not being accustomed to seeing her nipples stick out in front of her, which before surgery were lower on her breasts and less obvious.)

The Goins describe another patient who was forewarned about reduced breast and nipple sensation after surgery. Nevertheless, her first sexual encounter subsequent to her breast reduction was emotionally upsetting. When her partner caressed her breasts, she felt only pressure and no erotic sensation. She was shocked and became panicky. Jackie, whose experience with a breast lift and augmentation was reported earlier, relates her first post-surgery sexual experience:

> *Jackie.* We didn't have sex for about six weeks. I just didn't feel like it. When we finally did, I was self-conscious. I was afraid he wouldn't like them, even though he had seen and touched them while I was recuperating. My doctor had warned me about sensation loss. As it turned out, I still had some sensation, though not as much as before. We have a good sexual relationship, and the reduced sensation wasn't that important to me. I was pleased that he enjoyed my new breasts, and I felt good about myself.

Patients rarely discuss their uncomfortable feelings, fears, and anxieties after surgery for fear of being thought odd or strange. Some see admitting such feelings as a sign of weakness. Instead they may seek reassurance from their doctors about scars or skin discoloration, or they may talk to the doctor's nurse or staff.

Creating a Positive Body Image

Dissatisfaction with an aspect of physical appearance does not necessarily constitute a poor body image. Most people experience minor dissatisfactions at various times in their lives. A problem with body image exists when unhappiness reaches such a level that a person has trouble accepting his or her appearance, when the felt dissatisfaction interferes with the ability to have satisfactory relationships, or when the focus of energy is on being unhappy with some aspect of physical appearance. Fortunately, a negative body image can be overcome. Progress has been made in the assessment and treatment of body image disturbances,[19] and some therapists specialize in this type of treatment. An excellent self-help book is also available, *What Do You See When You Look in the Mirror,* by Thomas F. Cash, Ph.D.[20] In his book, Dr. Cash provides a body image self-test for assessing thoughts, feelings, and behaviors related to physical appearance, physical activities, and health. He subdivides body image into a number of components. The Body/Self Relationship Test and related Profile assess four of these components and are reprinted at the end of this chapter.

Section A of the test provides an Appearance Evaluation score that reveals the test taker's overall perception or "big picture." It is possible to be dissatisfied with one or a few aspects of appearance and yet be generally happy with overall appearance. A score in the average to very high range in this section points to a generally positive overall body image and suggests that any particular dissatisfactions are kept in perspective. A low score here suggests a possible body image disturbance. Unhappiness with one or more body parts may be contributing to an overall negative body image.

In section B, the Appearance Orientation score suggests the degree to which the test taker is invested in his or her appearance and how much appearance is emphasized over other qualities or traits. A score in the high or very high range indicates the test taker is very appearance oriented and may place too much importance on looks. If a great deal of time and energy is being spent in the pursuit of attractiveness, there may be too much emphasis on appearance. A high score in this section together with a low score in the Appearance Evaluation suggests that in spite of a considerable investment of time and energy, efforts are not paying off. There may be too much dependence on looks as a source of self-esteem. On the other hand, a very low score in this section could suggest that the test taker is discouraged or sees no point in trying to improve.

In section C, the Fitness/Health Orientation score suggests the degree of investment in something other than attractiveness. People who care about physical fitness and health, who exercise regularly and make healthy food choices, and who are health conscious, score higher in this category. A comparison of the score category (i.e., very low to very high) in this section to the score category in Section B provides a sense of relative investment in appearance to the investment in fitness/health. If the appearance orientation score category is high or very high and the fitness/health orientation score is low or very low, more energy needs to be put into efforts for physical well-being. Conversely, a high fitness/health orientation score and a low appearance orientation score may point to other problems, such as an eating disorder.

In section D, the Fitness/Health Evaluation score assesses the test taker's sense of being physically fit or unfit. High scorers regard themselves as physically fit, "in shape," healthy, or athletically active and competent. They experience their efforts to increase or maintain fitness and health as paying off. Low scorers feel physically unfit, "out of shape," unhealthy, or athletically unskilled. They need to find ways to strengthen and enjoy their physical well-being.

Complete the Body/Self Relationship Test that appears at the end of this chapter. Score yourself on each section and locate your score in the appropriate Profile. To assess your body image, review your scores in reference to the discussion of sections A, B, C, and D.

Overcoming a negative body image begins with identifying and verbalizing the shame that underlies the self-consciousness about a perceived personal deficit. When and how did the self-consciousness begin? What cultural, developmental, interpersonal, and emotional influences contributed to concern about appearance? After discerning the history of body image concerns, current situations that create anxiety or distress about appearance are considered—for example, wearing a bathing suit or seeing oneself in a mirror.

An important part of creating a positive body image is to change thinking. The discrepancy between the perceived self and the ideal self needs to be understood, and the reasonableness of the selected ideal must be challenged. One needs to reevaluate the perceived self, emphasizing the positive qualities, as opposed to the negatives. Critical and disparaging internal dialogues must be replaced by more positive thoughts. Counterarguments are generated to disputed irrational beliefs. Recognizing, challenging, disputing, and reconstructing negative thoughts is important. Using self-accepting and supportive private body talk is a key to creating a positive body image.

In addition to replacing negative thinking with positive body talk, one must learn to handle differently stress and situations that engender distress about appearance. One approach is to image encountering situations that evoke negative thoughts and feelings about the body and learn to cope better with them. Learning to elicit the relaxation response can be helpful. Combining relaxation with images of distressing body-image situations helps to desensitize reactions to such situations. Yet another approach is to learn to stand in front of a mirror and engage in positive or coping self-statements. Replacing avoidant body-image behaviors (for example, not wearing revealing clothes) and compulsive body-image rituals (for example, frequent mirror checking) with affirming activities, such as pursuing physical fitness through regular exercise is important. Working with a trained therapist who is experienced in working with body image issues can be very helpful in implementing these techniques.

Summary

Perceptions and mental pictures and attitudes, beliefs, thoughts, and feelings about the body constitute body image. Body image begins to develop in infancy and is influenced by the reactions of others and the individual's experiences over time, as well as in the context of a particular culture and historical period. The key to understanding motivation for and recovery from cosmetic surgery is body image. Dissatisfaction with an aspect of body image underlies the motivation for surgery and does not necessarily imply a significantly poor body image. A body image disturbance, which is a serious and debilitating problem, can lead a person to seek multiple surgeries and to find dissatisfaction with objectively good results. Psychological treatment can assist in the development of a more positive and healthy body image. A person with a positive body image may still choose to have cosmetic surgery for a perceived deficit in appearance and is more likely to have a positive outcome.

The Body/Self Relationship Test

How well does each statement describe you?

1 = Definitely Disagree; 2 = Mostly Disagree; 3 = Neither Agree Nor Disagree; 4 = Mostly Agree; 5 = Definitely Agree

_____ 1. My body is sexually appealing.

_____ 2. I like my looks just the way they are.

_____ 3. Most people would consider me good-looking.

_____ 4. I like the way I look without my clothes.

_____ 5. I like the way my clothes fit me.

_____ 6. I dislike my physique.

_____ 7. I am physically unattractive.

_____ 8. Before going out in public, I always notice how I look.

_____ 9. I am careful to buy clothes that will make me look my best.

_____ 10. I check my appearance in a mirror whenever I can.

_____ 11. Before going out, I usually spend a lot of time getting ready.

_____ 12. It is important that I always look good.

_____ 13. I am self-conscious if my grooming isn't right.

_____ 14. I take special care with my hair grooming.

_____15. I am always trying to improve my physical appearance.

_____16. I usually wear whatever is handy without caring how it looks.

_____17. I don't care what people think about my appearance.

_____18. I never think about my appearance.

_____19. I use very few grooming products.

_____20. I easily learn physical skills.

_____21. I am very well-coordinated.

_____22. I am in control of my health.

_____23. I am seldom physically ill.

_____24. From day to day, I never know how my body will feel.

_____25. I am a physically healthy person.

_____26. I would pass most physical-fitness tests.

_____27. My physical endurance is good.

_____28. My health is a matter of unexpected ups and downs.

_____29. I do poorly in physical sports or games.

_____30. I often feel vulnerable to sickness.

_____31. I know a lot about things that affect my physical health.

_____32. I have deliberately developed a healthy lifestyle.

_____33. Good health is one of the most important things in my life.

_____34. I don't do anything that I know might threaten my health.

_____35. I do things to increase my physical strength.

_____36. I often read books and magazines that pertain to health.

_____37. I work to improve my physical stamina.

_____38. I try to be physically active.

_____39. I know a lot about physical fitness.

_____40. Being physically fit is not a strong priority in my life.

_____41. I am not involved in a regular exercise program.

_____42. I take my health for granted.

_____43. I make no special effort to eat a balanced and nutritious diet.

_____44. I don't care to improve my abilities in physical activities.

Scoring Your Body/Self Relationship Test

This test is a little tricky to score. Because it is really four tests in one, you will calculate four separate scores. Also, due to the fact that some test items are worded positively and others are worded negatively, you must use the specific formulas given. Each formula requires that you sum ratings on particular items, subtract the sum of ratings on other items, then add a certain number of points. (Points are added to adjust for the wording of certain items.) Just follow the formulas and you will have your scores for the four subtests.

A. To determine your *Appearance Evaluation* score:

Step 1. Add your ratings on items 1-5.   _____

Step 2. Add your ratings on items 6-7.   _____

Step 3. Subtract the amount in Step 2 from
     the amount in Step 1.   _____

Step 4. Add 12 points to the Step 3 amount.   _____

                                                 + 12

Score =   _____

On the appropriate Profile enter the amount under "Score." Make sure it falls somewhere from 7 to 35. Mark the box for your score on the Profile grid.

B. To determine your *Appearance Orientation* score:

Step 1. Add your ratings on items 8-15.   _____

Step 2. Add your ratings on items 16-19.   _____

Step 3. Subtract the amount in Step 2 from
     the amount in Step 1.   _____

Step 4. Add 24 points to the Step 3 amount.   _____

                                                 + 24

Score =   _____

Enter the final amount on the appropriate Profile. It should fall somewhere between 12 and 60. Mark the correct box on the Profile.

C. To determine your *Fitness/Health Evaluation* score:

Step 1. Add your ratings on items 20-27. _____

Step 2. Add your ratings on items 28-30. _____

Step 3. Subtract the amount in Step 2 from the amount in Step 1. _____

Step 4. Add 18 points to the Step 3 amount. _____

+ 18

Score = _____

Enter the final amount on the appropriate Profile. Your score should be a number between 11 and 55. Mark the correct box on the appropriate Profile.

D. To determine your *Fitness/Health Orientation* score:

Step 1. Add your ratings on items 31-39. _____

Step 2. Add your ratings on items 40-44. _____

Step 3. Subtract the amount in Step 2 from the amount in Step 1. _____

Step 4. Add 30 points to the Step 3 amount. _____

+ 30

Score = _____

Enter the amount in Step 4 on the appropriate Profile. Your score should fall between 14 and 70. Mark the correct box on the Profile.

© Copyright 1995, Thomas F. Cash. Reprinted with permission from *What Do You See When You Look in the Mirror?*

The Personal Body-Image Profile for Women

Score the tests as explained earlier. Enter each test score in the blank provided below. Then, to classify your score from "Very Low" to "Very High," mark an X in the appropriate box on the Profile.

BODY-IMAGE TEST	Score	Very Low	Low	Average	High	Very High
A. Appearance Evaluation	_____	7-17	18-23	24-25	26-29	30-35
B. Appearance Orientation	_____	12-40	41-46	47-48	49-53	54-60

	Score	Very Low	Low	Average	High	Very High
C. Fitness/Health Evaluation	_____	11-33	34-40	41-42	43-47	48-55
D. Fitness/Health Orientation	_____	14-41	42-49	50-52	53-59	60-70

The Personal Body-Image Profile for Men

Score the tests as explained earlier. Enter each test score in the blank provided below. Then, to classify your score from "Very Low" to "Very High," mark an X in the appropriate box on the Profile.

BODY-IMAGE TEST	Score	Very Low	Low	Average	High	Very High
A. Appearance Evaluation	_____	7-19	20-24	25-26	27-29	30-35
B. Appearance Orientation	_____	12-36	37-42	43-44	45-50	51-60
C. Fitness/Health Evaluation	_____	11-36	37-42	43-44	45-50	51-55
D. Fitness/Health Orientation	_____	14-41	42-49	50-52	53-59	60-70

9

Your Nose Looks
Okay to Me

It had been three weeks since my surgery. Most of the swelling had gone down, but there were still some significant bruises under my eyes. The left side of my mouth didn't respond quite the same as my right, and sometimes when I spoke my speech was slurred. I had not yet ventured outside my home nor seen any of my friends. About this time, some friends called to invite my husband and me to a wine tasting sponsored by a local wine vendor. I wasn't sure I should go. (And I wasn't then aware that drinking alcohol causes temporary swelling and increases skin discomfort.) I hadn't been out in public yet, and I wasn't sure I was ready. I still couldn't get my contacts into my eyes, because the lids were too tender to touch. My glasses didn't fit my face any more because of residual swelling and because some large scars had emerged over my ears. I had to stretch my glasses to make them fit, and even then the pressure against the scars made me uncomfortable. Plus, the scars were itchy. I surveyed my bruises in the mirror. I thought I might be able to cover them with a concealer, and with enough make-up, maybe no one would notice.

I hadn't told Ginny and Richard about my operation, and when we met at the wine tasting, I pretended as if nothing had happened. I hoped they wouldn't notice, but the shock in their eyes when they saw me told me otherwise.

"How *are* you?" cooed Ginny, in her usual bubbly way.

"Fine," I responded curtly. Nothing more was said about me or my appearance, but the atmosphere that evening was strained.

A few days later, I called Ginny and acknowledged that indeed, I had had face-lift surgery.

"I wasn't going to say anything if you hadn't," said Ginny.

As the swelling and bruising subsided over time, my new face began to emerge. I looked different to me, and I looked different to my friends. Everyone exclaimed how much younger I looked. Many months after surgery, a good friend confided that she had great difficulty putting together my new face with the voice she knew. It took being together again several times, she said, for her to feel that I was still the friend she used to know. My sister later told me that when she first saw me several days after surgery she was startled and upset, though she concealed it. She was afraid I wouldn't fully recover. My husband, too, maintained a cheerful and positive front for the first few weeks, only to tell me later how worried he had been when I first came home. I was not aware of these reactions of family and friends until much, much later.

Traditional rules of etiquette don't help other people know what to say to someone who has had cosmetic surgery. Not only does no one know how to deal with such awkward situations, cosmetic surgery patients often don't know who to tell or when to tell them. Most people who undergo some cosmetic surgery procedure are hesitant to reveal this to others, or they have a great deal of ambivalence in doing so. Jackie reported that on the one hand, she was upset when her friends didn't comment or ask to see her newly done breasts, but on the other hand she was glad they didn't.

Breast augmentation patients tend to be more open about their surgery than patients who get another cosmetic procedure. These patients are often quite happy to have "after" pictures taken by their surgeons and are frequently willing to let friends see, too. One woman who had breast augmentation enthusiastically encouraged friends to feel as well as view her new bosom. Her friends were understandably perplexed by her offer.

When to go out in public or appear at a social event is an individual decision. Myrna, a business woman, arranged time off for her classic face-lift and eyelid operation but could not reschedule one of her important clients. She had to keep their appointment just a few days after surgery, so she forewarned the client that she would be wearing bandages around her head and face and would probably look "funny." The client apparently took it in stride. In contrast to Myrna's assertive stance, another woman kept herself housebound for six weeks until she felt okay about being seen in public. Paulette went to the store a week after her nose surgery, proudly wearing a small bandage over her nose, knowing she had at last realized her dreams of a better-looking nose.

Some who have cosmetic surgery decide to say little or nothing to others about their surgery, regarding this as a private matter. Jackie explained to her 25-year-old son (who lived with her and Tony) that she had had "female surgery," but provided no further explanation. When Carole remarried, she simply didn't tell her new husband that her beautiful breasts were partly man-made. Anita never told her parents she had her breasts augmented because she was afraid they might feel they failed in some way to raise her "right." One husband and wife each had face-lifts at the same time, but when he told his good friend about their surgeries she was furious he had revealed something so personal. A common reaction of others is to notice that something is different but not know exactly what it is. They may make comments such as, "You look different. Did you lose weight or do something new with your hair?" The cosmetic surgery patient must address the question: Who do I tell, and when do I tell them? Shame and guilt over having such surgery is common and is stimulated by the social taboos that still influence attitudes about cosmetic surgery.

Social Taboos and Cosmetic Surgery

"How could you even think about letting yourself get carved up just to look better?"

"Why can't you accept what God intended for you?"

"Why would you want to do such a thing? You look fine as you are."

"Do you realize what the money you are spending for cosmetic surgery could buy?"

"How could you consider treating your body so recklessly? What if something goes wrong?"

"Don't you realize you are capitulating to a system that victimizes women by convincing them that young and beautiful is what really counts?"

Those not yet faced with the ravages of aging or who are more accepting of physical imperfections easily find reasons why not to get cosmetic surgery. They may disdain another's wish to slow the aging process or to alter a perceived deficit and righteously assert, "I would never have cosmetic surgery." Even though more and more people have a favorable opinion about cosmetic surgery, some reactions range from incredulousness and outright disbelief that such an idea could be entertained to thinly-veiled criticisms, hostility, and even adamant disapproval. No wonder that talking to others about cosmetic surgery is done with trepidation.

The social taboos and prohibitions that have kept cosmetic surgery in the closet for so long spring from a variety of perspectives. Many people feel that self-imposed surgery to change appearance is a vain, superficial, narcissistic, and unrealistic search for youth and the approval of others. Surgery to repair damage from a car accident or to reconstruct a breast after cancer may be permissible, but not surgery for the sole purpose of enhancing appearance. Not only is the latter unthinkable, to many it is worthy of condemnation.

Despite society's increasingly positive view of cosmetic surgery, acceptance within the Judeo-Christian heritage is still lagging. Some believe it is not right to modify what God, fate, or genetic inheritance has provided. Those who are beautiful from birth have been favored by God. The rest should accept their fate and go forward from there. To desire more than God or fate has given is vain and invites God's reprisals. Suffering a horrible complication of cosmetic surgery could be a punishment if such vanity is indulged. Such fears of celestial reprisal are evidence of the deep-felt guilt instilled by this heritage. Condemnation of elective surgery is reasonable and appropriate to those who hold these views. Little or no emotional support is likely to be provided to loved ones or friends who want cosmetic surgery for "vain" reasons, rather than because of a life-threatening disease or to correct a congenital disfigurement.

Others are more pragmatic in their assessment of the validity of cosmetic surgery. One well-known plastic surgeon, whose specialty is the reconstruction of ears damaged by accident or by birth defect, holds great disdain for his colleagues who "squander" their talents performing "mere" cosmetic surgery. Waste is the issue for him, and many others share his perspective. With so much illness in the world and so many people that have "real" medical problems, they argue, the diversion of resources to cosmetic enhancement is unjustified. This view presupposes the existence of an objective standard that can establish "need" and prioritize which needs will be met in service of the greater good. Elective surgery, of course, would be low on the list, if not eliminated all together.

Similarly, pragmatism may be the standard applied within the family. Some family members object to another's wish for cosmetic surgery, arguing that the money could be used for a better purpose. Surgery for cosmetic purposes is almost never covered by insurance, and its cost must be covered out of pocket. When limited funds are committed for one person's benefit, another family member can become jealous or resentful that they are not getting their fair share of family resources.

Feminists are also vocal in their condemnation of cosmetic surgery, which they see as voluntary and unnecessary mutilation in response to social pressure. They argue that women who get cosmetic surgery are not acting autonomously, but are coerced into such surgery by media (mis)representation and a male-dominated "system" in which men control women by convincing them that beauty is the only real measure of their self-worth. By submitting to cosmetic surgery, women capitulate to the oppressor. In *Lear's* magazine Margaret Morganroth Gullette exhorts women (and men) to "resist" and to believe "You're beautiful as you are."[1] In particular, Gullette indicts doctors who publish self-endorsements and sell cosmetic surgery by convincing people, especially women, that they are "ugly and wrong."

In a complementary article in *Lear's*, Carol Isaak Barden writes that she, too, felt it wasn't right to mess with Mother Nature.[2] Her attitude began to change, however, when her own face started to go south. "The bags under my eyes, and my heavy eyelids, made me downright cranky; even after a good night's rest I looked half asleep." The very thought of having her eyes done filled her feminist heart with guilt. She reminded herself that women shouldn't give in to such vanity—her mother didn't. Besides, something could go wrong, leaving her blind or scarred for life. Still, there was that face in the mirror. She was a woman who took pride in her appearance, thinking nothing of waiting in line to get her hair done or her nails lacquered. She exercised and watched her diet to stay trim, and she got regular facials and massages. When she told her best friend she was thinking of getting a face-lift, her friend gasped, "You? Exactly what is the problem?" implying the existence of some unresolved issues in her life. Another friend responded, "Why would you want to risk death? It's a side effect, you know. The doctor could botch it and you might look worse, not better." Yet another commented, "People are so into themselves!"

As Marcia and John Goin point out, those who are relatively unconcerned about their appearance often find it difficult to comprehend the desire to have a face-lift, breast augmentation, nose reshaping, or some other surgery to change or improve appearance.[3] In all likelihood, they have not thought much about the intimate connection between the sense of self and feelings about one's body. They may be young or without blemish and have not felt the sting of a perceived deficit. Or they see cultural influences, fashion, the media, or "the system" as culprits that create and promote images of "the beautiful people." They decry the beauty-is-good stereotype and cite social factors as the impetus that drives people (mostly women) to have cosmetic surgery.

Unfortunately, the social taboos that deny cosmetic surgery as an option fail to account for the benefits it can have on the psyche and self-esteem. Carol Isaak Barden described herself as feeling more self-assured after surgery. She termed it "life affirming." Ultimately, the choice to have cosmetic surgery is a personal one that is made in the context of a cultural and social milieu.

Social Context of Cosmetic Surgery

The social context of cosmetic surgery has been largely ignored, both by writers and by the few scientists who study the effects of cosmetic surgery on patients. As noted in Chapter 2, the reactions of significant others affect the person anticipating or recovering from cosmetic surgery more so than do the reactions of strangers. Ideally, family, friends, and co-workers understand the desire to have surgery and give the patient support and positive feedback afterward. With support and reinforcement patients should become more socially relaxed and poised. Unfortunately, this is not always the case.

Frequently, friends or family members are critical of the desire to have cosmetic surgery, and this bias does not disappear after surgery is over. Prospective patients need to prepare for this kind of reaction.

Caroline Cline, M.D., a plastic surgeon in San Francisco, prepares her patients by asking them who they've told about their planned surgery and how they will deal with criticism from others. She asks her patients to consider how their mother is likely to react to the patient's wish for surgery, how Dad will feel, and what friends will say. She may ask, "What's the worst thing a friend could say to you after surgery?" These questions are intended to get the patient to think about and prepare for the reactions of others.

Reactions of Others Before Surgery

The reactions of friends to the idea of getting cosmetic surgery are often experienced as undermining or unsupportive. When Paulette confided to a friend that she was thinking of undergoing surgery to reshape her nose, her friend responded as many do in such circumstances, "Your nose looks okay to me." Though possibly well-meant, the remark was nonetheless perplexing. Was her friend being disingenuous to avoid appearing critical, or was she implying that Paulette was vain?

Sometimes people are negative about cosmetic surgery because it seems selfish and vain. Others may interpret the desire for surgery as a reinforcement of the male tendency to view women as sex objects or as submitting to male-defined ideals for women. Family members may see the wish to change an inherited feature as a personal rejection. Spouses may view the desire for cosmetic surgery as a potential threat to the relationship. Sometimes, the only source of supportive comments is from others who have had cosmetic surgery.

The Spouse Who Says No

A red flag for many plastic surgeons is the spouse who is adamantly opposed to his or her partner's cosmetic surgery. Theoretically and legally, a mentally competent adult can decide whether to have an operation. In reality, the current or potential reaction of a significant other plays an important role for both the patient and the surgeon. Usually it is the husband who strongly disapproves of his wife's desire to change her nose, get a face-lift, or reduce the size of her breasts. To the extent that a wife experiences a feature as displeasing, the negative impact on her self-esteem may be an important factor in the power balance in the marriage. A woman with poor self-esteem can be more easily exploited, consciously or unconsciously, by her husband.

One study investigated the psychological aspects of breast reconstruction after mastectomy from the husband's standpoint.[4] Most of the respondents were white, highly educated, and from high income groups. Although only a small proportion of questionnaires were returned, the results were surprising and unexpected. Only 20 percent of the husbands were somewhat in favor of breast reconstruction, 33 percent were neutral, 7 percent were mildly opposed, and 27 percent were strongly opposed. Thus, more than a third were against breast reconstruction after mastectomy!

The results also indicated that the women who had breast reconstruction were more likely to have a good recovery from mastectomy if their husbands were involved and supportive. When the husband was involved in the decision-making process about treatment of breast cancer, visited the hospital frequently, resumed sexual relations early after surgery, and was willing to look at the woman's operative site after surgery, the woman generally made a good post-operative adjustment. It seems reasonable to assume, based on these results, that when spouses and significant others are involved and supportive, patients recover better and more quickly from any cosmetic surgery.

Although most of the husbands surveyed coped well with their spouse's surgery, a small subgroup became distressed at the time of the operation, remained distressed, and reported deterioration of their marital relationship over time. Although usually the surgeon was seen as an ally, some husbands saw the surgeon as an adversary, calling him a "butcher" or "sadistic." In some cases, a surgeon-husband-wife triangle developed, in which the husband claimed that the wife now hated him instead of the doctor who "mutilated" her. In light of these reactions, surgeons are understandably hesitant to operate when a spouse opposes surgery.

Nonsupport from Family and Friends

Parents and other family members may oppose surgery, especially if the feature to be changed is an indicator of ethnicity or is a family characteristic. Some family members may feel that the patient is getting too much of scarce family resources, money, attention, and leave from his or her usual duties. A parent's desire for cosmetic surgery can raise issues about aging and dying for children, because such surgery reminds them that they too are getting older.

Friends and co-workers may also be less than supportive. As with a spouse, appearance can play a role in the balance of power between friends. A change in appearance of one person may imply that the rules of the relationship are up for renegotiation. When one person increases his or her physical attractiveness through cosmetic surgery, the other person in the relationship can feel "one down" and less valued. Knowing this intuitively, if not consciously, friends may actively discourage pursuit of cosmetic surgery.

Reactions of Others in Early Recovery

Sometimes family members and friends are mostly curious about the patient's cosmetic surgery. Myrna said her parents and friends mainly wanted to know how it felt and when the stitches would come out. Anita tried to camouflage her newly augmented breasts by initially wearing large, flowing blouses in order to ease the transition to a new public image, but when her best friend came to visit a few weeks after surgery, she cried out, "Oh my God, where did you get those?"

Sometimes, family members have other reactions. When John first saw his wife after breast reduction surgery, he was upset. "I didn't know if she would ever be okay again. She looked terrible. I didn't want her to do it in the first place, and when she went ahead anyway I was really angry with her." Family members may withhold their approval not because they are hostile, but because they are cautious or bewildered. Initially, they may hesitate to be enthusiastic because they are unsure of the results and frightened for the welfare of the patient. When the patient is swollen and bruised, family members don't know what to make of it. Any operation creates stress for family members, who worry about the patient's well-being. This is exacerbated if the patient complains of pain, becomes depressed, or suffers complications. If a family member were initially opposed to the surgery, he may now turn hostile.

During the first few weeks after surgery, the cosmetic surgery patient is especially vulnerable to the comments of others. At this time, the final results are often not fully discernible because of swelling and bruising, and patients are usually dependent on others to some extent to get their physical and emotional needs met. If those providing immediate care think cosmetic surgery is frivolous, or if they disapprove in some way, their judgments are likely to be conveyed, even if subtly, to the patient. In early recovery, the patient is likely to have fewer resources for coping with a lack of support. Because her energy is low at this time, the patient may not be able to deal with the distressing situations that she was previously able to manage, such as an unhappy relationship, a difficult child, or a stressful job.

After surgery, it is not uncommon for a husband to joke that his wife might leave him for a younger man, now that she looks younger herself. Although this may sound possessive, it reflects his emotional attachment to her and his latent anxiety that this change threatens the relationship. If this anxiety is not allayed, it can create stress, which might be expressed as jealousy or possessiveness. This may have been the basis for the comment Tony made to Jackie several months after her breast lift and augmentation: "I bet your next husband will like your boobs."

Adult children can also react negatively to a parent's cosmetic surgery. For many children, no matter what their age, having a mother suddenly looking younger or different is threatening. The change can awaken conflicts or needs from the past. One such example is that of a patient who came to the doctor's office four days after a face-lift accompanied by her son, who was in his late 20s. The son looked hostile. In the son's presence, the patient said to the surgeon, "He's angry I had this done." Her son defended himself by saying that he opposed the unnecessary risks this type of elective procedure entailed. The patient later told her surgeon in confidence that while the ostensible reason was true, her son had told her, "Without your big double chin, you don't look like Grandma, and I used to snuggle up against her neck while I was young."

Family and friends can help by simply listening nonjudgmentally to the patient's concerns. Often patients feel guilty about not being able to take care of themselves or not being able to bounce back as quickly as they thought they would. Feeling down, blue, or somewhat depressed after surgery is fairly common. Giving advice and telling the patient she shouldn't feel "that way" should be avoided. Reassuring the patient that the physical trauma and discomfort will pass in time and encouraging her to talk about her feelings is the best comfort that can be given.

How the cosmetic surgery patient handles unsympathetic remarks by family or friends also makes a difference. Cleo's mother brought her home from her face lift surgery because Cleo's husband Dave was out of town on business during her surgery. When Dave returned the next day, he took one look at Cleo's swollen and bruised face and recoiled in horror. "You are grotesque! You look hideous! How could you do this to me?" Dave stormed out of the house, leaving Cleo in tears. A few hours later the phone rang. It was the wife of a couple who were mutual friends. She told Cleo that Dave had come to their home feeling very upset and remorseful for his reaction to Cleo's appearance. The friend suggested that Dave stay at their place the night and return home the following day. The next evening Cleo was prepared for Dave's return. Although her face was still swollen and bruised, she dressed herself in her sexiest negligee and plumped up the pillows on her bed. Then she took a took a large, brown grocery bag and cut out two eyes, drew a happy face on the bag, and propped herself up in the bed. When she heard Dave come in the door, she put the bag over her head. He came into the bedroom without looking at her and began putting down his keys and other items. "I'm sorry about what I said," he offered. Suddenly he seemed to catch a glimpse of something out of the corner of his eye. He spun around and saw Cleo sitting among the pillows, wearing her sexiest best with a brown bag over her head. Dave broke up with laughter, and the difficulties created dissipated. Cleo had managed to defuse a potentially painful problem with humor.

Reactions of Others in Later Recovery

Reportedly, Donald Trump said he hated touching "those plastic things" after his wife Ivana had breast augmentation. Other men are delighted at the newfound eroticism that breast augmentation can bring to a relationship. Anita, who was unmarried at the time of her breast augmentation, talked about how surgery changed her relationships with men: "When men would meet me they would often say, 'Oh, the first thing that attracted me to you was your beautiful breasts.' That would create a lot of conflict in me. I would think, if they had met me before surgery, I wonder what they would have been attracted to then. Before surgery I hadn't had that much sexual experience, but after the breast surgery I seemed to have a lot more men interested in me sexually. They would focus on my breasts and say things like, 'I just love your breasts. You could be in *Playboy*.' It seemed to me that all they could see were my breasts, and they never noticed the real me."

After the bruising and swelling have diminished, the reactions of others can still be surprising. One woman, who prior to her rhinoplasty and face-lift had been close friends with a glamorous neighbor, found the neighbor no longer had time for her. A partner who may have been very supportive and in favor of the surgery beforehand may turn suddenly irritable and distant. Those who think the patient is trying to deny his ethnic or cultural heritage may be critical or rejecting.

The reactions of others affect how the patient feels about her surgery. Youngsters are very sensitive to the reactions of a parent, especially the mother, and to the reactions of friends and peers. Often, friends of an adolescent are more supportive of surgical results than are friends of the middle-aged woman who gets cosmetic surgery.[5] Adult women are especially vulnerable to the opinions of their friends, more so those to that of their husbands. Just at the time she needs their support the most, friends may consciously or unconsciously make unkind remarks that can undermine the patient, such as: "After seeing what you look like, I'd never have it done." "Gee, you sure are swollen." "Your eyes don't match." "How come Betty looks so much better than you do? She went to the same surgeon." "Do you realize you could have bought a new car for what that cost you?"

Unkind remarks may be prompted by a variety of causes. They may derive from jealousy and resentment that the patient is attempting to look more attractive. A friend may wish she had the money or the courage to have the operation herself. The person making the remark may fear that the patient will no longer value him or her and may replace their relationship with another one. Criticism may be intended to devalue the patient and enhance the critic. Anita recalled a painful incident that happened to her: "One of my co-workers called me aside one day and said, 'Did you know that the bimbo secretary has been telling everyone that you've had a boob job?' I was stunned and hurt. I found the opportunity a little later to confront her. 'Who do you think you are talking about me behind my back? You have no right to delve into my personal business.' Apparently she was pretty frightened because I never heard anything more, but the incident made me feel vulnerable to other people's nastiness."

Many times hurtful remarks are unexpected and can come from surprising sources. Jackie was away on a business trip and having breakfast in the hotel restaurant. Seated at the next table were several men who had obviously been out on the town the previous night. One men remarked to the others, "Did you catch that blond last night?" Another man replied, "You mean the surgically enhanced one, the one with the bolt-ons?" All the men laughed.

Although the remark was not directed at Jackie, she felt humiliated. Later, she reflected on the contradiction inherent in breast-enhancement surgery: beautiful breasts are the focus of much attention, especially from men, and highly valued in this society. Women without beautiful breasts can be derided by terms such as "droopy tits," "knee knockers," and "fried eggs." Yet having beautiful breasts, even if they are God given, exposes a woman to the assumption that she has had surgical enhancement. Actually having such surgery prompts additional criticism and ridicule because they are "fake." (Many of these same men would wear a hair piece, get a hair transplant, or comb thinning hair to camouflage baldness.)

Not only can others say things that are hurtful or unsupportive, cosmetic surgery patients may be surprised by what others do. Jackie was dumbfounded when Tony's old friend from out of town greeted her by grabbing both of her breasts and squeezing. It was as if he regarded her breasts as objects to fondle rather than a part of her body. Would he have done this had her breasts been natural, instead of surgically enhanced?

Another woman who had a breast augmentation was horrified when a co-worker to whom she had casually confided that her breasts were "paid for" announced it at the dinner table to the rest of their co-workers. The woman with the breast augmentation was angry with herself for giving out such personal information. Would the co-worker have made an announcement if she had a gall bladder operation instead? Why would the co-worker assume she had the right to relate something so personal? It seems that cosmetic surgery, and breast surgery in particular, can be titillating and shocking. If cosmetic surgery patients are unprepared for hurtful remarks and actions, they are likely to feel confused and angry when it happens. The best defense is to be forewarned and have a response prepared.

Summary

The social context of cosmetic surgery has been largely neglected in research, and most of the information in this regard comes from anecdotal and clinical sources. Social taboos continue to keep the desire for and the obtaining of cosmetic surgery "in the closet." Proscriptions related to vanity, morals, and pragmatism as well as concerns about the oppression of women keep taboos in place. Those who seek and obtain cosmetic surgery are vulnerable to the opinions and actions of significant others, who often make unkind remarks, either consciously or unconsciously. In fact, cosmetic surgery patients need the emotional support of others, especially in the early recovery stage, the first few months after surgery. Those who get this support have a better and faster recovery than those who do not. When support from the social milieu is not provided, the patient needs to obtain it elsewhere. The services of a psychotherapist may be needed if other sources are not adequate or available.

10

I Like How I Look, But . . .

After several months, my bruises had disappeared and most of the noticeable swelling was gone. I was alarmed because the scars over and behind my ears had gotten large and lumpy, a condition known as hypertrophy. My doctor injected cortisone to help reduce the size of the scars and instructed me to massage them regularly. He indicated that in a few more months the scars would recede considerably. People do not realize that scarring is an inevitable consequence of most cosmetic procedures. Nor do they appreciate how long recovery really takes.

In contrast to some face-lift operations which can leave scars in front of the ears, the technique my doctor used hid the scars inside my ears. However, in the process my earlobes were permanently displaced. The pierced earring holes in my earlobes were now too close to my head. This complication was totally unanticipated by me but apparently was not a surprise to my doctor. He advised that in a few months I could have my earlobes re-pierced, but for now to wear clip-on earrings. (Some months later, when I attempted to have my earlobes re-pierced, hypertrophic scars formed around the new piercings, and I had to abandon the new earring holes.)

Hair loss along the hairline is another common complication of a face-lift and neck-lift. This problem was initially apparent at the back of my head, but within two to three months it had begun to correct itself and eventually grew back completely. At first I was self-conscious about this situation, which gave my hairline a strange look. But I had other things to be concerned about. More distressing was the prolonged loss of sensation in my cheek and neck region, as well as across the top of my scalp. Gradually, over the next year, sensation returned, but accompanied by itching. (Nevertheless, I consider myself fortunate; some people have permanent numbness or even pain.) Putting on makeup was a disconcerting experience for several months. A cinched up feeling under my chin and over the top of my head persisted for well over a year, and a tight sensation was still quite noticeable to me years later. This was a constant reminder that I had caused my body to be altered—and I was responsible for this discomfort.

Patient Satisfaction

Despite difficulties in recovery, most patients are satisfied with the results of cosmetic surgery. Satisfaction rates vary depending on the operation performed, how long after the operation satisfaction is assessed, and whether the patient is male or female. Generally males are more dissatisfied than females with the results of surgery. Some studies show that satisfaction with surgery increases over time.[1] Other studies suggest it decreases.[2]

One report reviewed eleven studies of patient satisfaction with various types of cosmetic surgery operations, including three studies of rhinoplasty operations, three of breast augmentation operations, two of face-lift operations, one of breast reduction, and two others. Satisfaction rates were assessed from 6 months to 17 years later and ranged from 65 percent (for males undergoing rhinoplasty) to 96 percent (on one study of rhinoplasty and one of mammaplasty)[3] The highest rate of post-operative dissatisfaction in the studies reviewed was 13 percent in a study of breast augmentation.[4]

Another study surveyed 1,000 patients who were 90 percent female and had a variety of cosmetic surgery operations and found an overall satisfaction rate of 81 percent. Seven percent complained that the operation did not fulfill their expectations and 12 percent said they looked better but didn't feel better about themselves after surgery.[5] Clearly, the majority of patients are satisfied with the *results* of cosmetic surgery, though such surgery may not always fulfill patients' wishes.

Although research is limited, satisfaction with specific operations varies. Some research has investigated patient satisfaction with eyelid surgery, liposuction procedures, face-lift operations, nose reshaping, and breast reduction.

Satisfaction with Eyelid Surgery

In 1992, eyelid surgery was the most frequently performed operation for women. Only recently has patient satisfaction with surgery on eyelids been assessed. In a study of patients who had either eyelid surgery for cosmetic reasons or to correct a minor functional problem, 55 percent of patients rated the results of surgery as the most important factor determining their satisfaction.[6] Other factors contributing to satisfaction included communication between the patient and the surgeon and his staff, the amount of pain and discomfort experienced, and the cost of the operation. Patients were happiest with the level of communication with the surgeon before and at the time of surgery, but they were dissatisfied with the falloff in communication after surgery. Patients were more concerned with the pain and discomfort experienced, both during and after surgery, than their surgeons realized. However, patients either did not tell their doctors, or they mentioned it only to the doctors' staff. Despite having some complaints, 80 percent of patients said they would recommend the procedure to a close friend or relative.

Satisfaction with Liposuction

In 1992 liposuction was the third most frequently performed cosmetic surgery procedure, constituting 12 percent of all such procedures done, and the second most frequently performed operation on women.[7] Since its introduction in the United States in 1982 liposuction has been increasingly refined and improved. Generally, patients are very satisfied and have few complaints.[8] One study of 2,009 patients who obtained one or more liposuction procedures between 1984 and 1989 assessed patients' experiences within one year of surgery.[9] Overall satisfaction was 88 percent, with females more satisfied than males. Only 3.4 percent reported being dissatisfied. The least satisfied were patients under the age of 20 or over the age of 60, and men were three times more likely to be unhappy with results than women. (However, a small percentage of female respondents said they didn't know if they were satisfied, and it is possible they were indeed dissatisfied but didn't want to say so.) Patients in this study most commonly complained that not enough fat had been removed. Overall, the most frequently reported undesired physical results included skin irregularities, swelling, and pigmentation changes.

A subsequent study investigated the experiences of over 1,000 lipectomy patients three years or more after surgery.[10] By this time, the satisfaction rate had fallen to 76 percent, with 6 percent saying they were dissatisfied. Older patients tended to be less satisfied. Males continued to be more dissatisfied than females, though to a lesser extent than they were immediately after surgery. Several years later, 54 percent said they would consider having liposuction again, and 31 percent said "perhaps." Those who were not sure had suffered considerable fatigue and found themselves unable to engage in their usual activities for a period of time after surgery. Only 8 percent said "definitely no," most often because they had experienced unexpected and unsatisfactory results. They complained that the surgery was too painful and uncomfortable afterwards, they didn't like having to wear the restrictive compression garments, and they were not willing to endure the fatigue and restricted physical activity levels that can accompany liposuction.

Liposuction is performed on different locations of the body, and satisfaction differs depending on location. Women are happiest with liposuction done on the abdomen and thighs. Dissatisfaction is highest when liposuction is done on the buttocks. The results of this study again confirmed that most complaints about liposuction, regardless of location, are that not enough fat is removed or the skin is left with a corrugated look. In nearly a third of all procedures, patients felt that not enough fat was removed, though they were generally still pleased with the results. Fewer than 3 percent of the procedures are associated with too much fat removal, which usually leads to dissatisfaction with the results. Sometimes when liposuction involves two sides of the body, both thighs or both arms, for example, more fat is removed from one side than the other. Although this would seem to be cause for upset, half of the patients who had asymmetrical results were still very happy. Even patients who experience some regrowth of fat, approximately 62 percent of liposuction patients, tend to be happy with their surgery.

Satisfaction with Face-Lift Surgery

Although face-lift surgery was only the fourth most frequently done operation on women in 1992 and the fifth most frequently done on men, most patient satisfaction research has focused on this type of surgery. Early studies of face-lift surgery failed to assess patient satisfaction. One of the first that did was a 1977 Mayo Clinic study that surveyed patients who had face-lift operations from 1962 to 1973. It found that nearly 13 percent said they were dissatisfied with their operation. Some of the reasons they gave for this were that they did not observe as much improvement as they expected, the results were not long lasting, or they thought it was not worth the cost. Of note is the fact that respondents in this study had had their operations several years before the study was done.

A study published in 1980 used both questionnaires and a structured interview to assess the responses of 50 female patients to face-lift surgery.[11] In their questionnaires, 60 percent rated their results as excellent and another 38 percent rated them good. In the interview with the psychiatrist, who was one of the researchers, the excellent rating fell to 54 percent and the good rating rose to 40 percent. No one rated their results as poor. Similarly an earlier study assessed 64 face-lift patients at Johns Hopkins Hospital 2 to 12 years after their operations, and again 60 percent rated their results as excellent.[12]

Satisfaction with Nose Reshaping

In 1992 nose reshaping was the most frequently performed operation for men seeking cosmetic surgery and the fifth most frequently done operation for women. Satisfaction rates for rhinoplasties ranged from a low of 65 percent to a high of 98 percent of patients who evaluated their results as either excellent or good. An early study of 300 patients who had a cosmetic rhinoplasty found that nearly 96 percent were satisfied with their surgical results.[13] In a more recent study of 103 women and 18 men who had rhinoplasties, 52 percent rated their surgical results as excellent and 44 percent rated them as good.[14] Only 1 percent said the results were poor. In describing the surgical results obtained, 90 percent said the changes were what they wanted and 10 percent said the results obtained were not what they expected. In another study of 98 women and 104 men undergoing rhinoplasty, 85 percent of women were satisfied six months after surgery, but this dropped to 68 percent three years later.[15] Eighty-six percent of men were initially satisfied, and 65 percent were still satisfied years later. A much smaller study of 15 women and 5 men with an average age of 23 found that 90 percent were either moderately or greatly pleased with results three months after surgery.[16] Ninety-one percent of 11 other rhinoplasty patients reported this level of satisfaction two years later.

Satisfaction with Breast Reduction

Patients who have breast reductions are among the most satisfied of all cosmetic surgery patients. Earlier studies of breast reduction surgery performed in Germany and elsewhere have found a high degree of patient satisfaction, usually in the range of 80 percent.[17] A more recent study reviewed long-term patient satisfaction using one of several breast reduction techniques more commonly used in the United States.[18] After surgery, 86 percent of patients were pleased with their new breast size, whereas 8 percent complained that their breasts had not been reduced enough. Eighty-three percent were pleased with the shape of their breasts, but 10 percent were not. More than three-fourths agreed that their breasts were of equal size, but 18 percent complained that their breasts were now asymmetrical. Sixty percent of patients reported a change in nipple sensation. In response to the question, Would you do it again? 94 percent said they would.

This research found that the most common physical symptoms prompting requests for breast reduction surgery were neck and back pain, posture problems, shoulder grooving from bra straps, pain in the breast, and skin rash under the breasts. Patients also complained about poor self-image, difficulty buying good-fitting clothing, and difficulty participating in sports. More than 90 percent reported that the surgery alleviated these symptoms.

Complications and Unmet Expectations

Satisfaction with the results of cosmetic surgery does not mean the patient has no complaints. The 1977 Mayo Clinic study of 324 patients who had undergone face-lifts several years earlier, mostly in the 1960s, revealed that 40 percent had some sort of complaint about the operation.[19] Generally, these included complaints of scarring, permanent numbness, and hair loss. Complete recovery from cosmetic surgery usually takes several months and some-times a year or more, depending on what is done. Even then, "complete re-covery" is a relative term. Complications of surgery can persist for months and in some cases can be permanent. One face-lift patient interviewed for this book complained that her hairline receded significantly on one side only and several years later had not regenerated; she is unable to comb her hair in certain styles. She rated her goals for surgery as only "partially met" but said that even so, she would do it again.

> *Paulette.* It took about a year for Paulette's nose to take final shape after her rhinoplasty, and she was very happy with the results. However, she developed a stuffy feeling in her head accompanied by sniffling. The breathing difficulty was variously attributed to an allergy, sinuses, or unidentified causes. Paulette admitted she wasn't sure the breathing problem was caused by the surgery but said she is so pleased with her appearance that she would do it again, even though it meant having to tolerate the breathing problem.

Anita experienced both physical problems and emotional reactions to her two breast augmentation surgeries:

> *Anita.* "Early on I really loved my new breasts, but then I started having some minor physical problems, and I kept thinking 'My natural breasts wouldn't do this.' I developed capsular contraction, and the way the surgeon would fix it was to manipulate the breasts and crush them. Not only did it hurt, but I was bothered by the "popping" sound. In addition, they would get very, very swollen around the time I was getting my period, to the point that I couldn't sleep on my stomach. Then there were times when I missed being the way I had been. I would miss being able to wear a nice pair of jeans with just a little T-shirt without a bra and look a little boyish and flat-chested. After the surgery I could not wear certain clothes because it would draw just an enormous amount of attention. I'm normally an outgoing person and pretty comfort-able in social situations, but having large breasts made me the focus of too much attention. Even after I had them replaced with smaller implants, I still felt uncomfortable. Unlike the first set of implants, the second set were sore all the time. I had to be careful hugging anyone or doing aerobics. Sleeping was often a problem because they were so tender. I developed a love/hate relationship with the second set, and eventually I decided they weren't worth it."

The "Ugly Duckling" Phenomenon

Sometimes patients must deal with unexpected emotional turmoil when cosmetic surgery triggers unanticipated behavioral changes. A patient who undergoes a type-changing operation may develop the "ugly duckling" phenomenon. Having been transformed into a "lovely swan," the patient faces new and unfamiliar experiences that can unleash behaviors formerly held in check. Those who were once shy and inhibited because of their appearance find themselves suddenly attractive, with new self-confidence and self-esteem. Sometimes patients act out and engage in uncharacteristic sexual experimentation, promiscuous behavior, or even precipitous marriages.[20] Interpersonal conflict may arise and result in marital distress, possibly even separation or divorce. If such patients become more assertive, they must also cope with the changed response of others to their new, more confident and assertive selves. This can cause problems. Like the adolescent who tests limits and has to learn to deal with his or her emerging sexuality and success and rejection, the "swan" may find herself in over her head at times. Psychotherapy can be helpful in learning to cope.[21] Over time, most patients adjust to the results and are pleased with the outcome.[22]

Depressive Reactions

As discussed in Chapter 7, depression is a common complication accompanying surgery of any kind. Usually depressive reactions to cosmetic surgery are mild and temporary. Feeling "down" or "blue" either immediately after the operation or a few weeks later occurs fairly often, in 25 to 60 percent of patients. Usually these mild symptoms are related to the aftereffects of anesthesia, pain, and trauma and abate in a few weeks as physical recovery proceeds. Sometimes depression continues much longer or is more intense, even leading to psychotic decompensation or suicide in rare cases. These more severe reactions may be the result of a preexisting but masked depression or a long-standing depression that has become part of the patient's character. A person trying to cope with a midlife crisis by getting cosmetic surgery may fall into a deep or long-lasting depression when surgery doesn't change her feelings. One widow who had not fully faced the implications of her husband's death became increasingly depressed after her face-lift, which did not correct the underlying loneliness and fear that her new circumstances as a widow brought. Although she was not fully conscious of it, her hope was that a face-lift would help attract a new mate and reinstate her emotional security.

Scarring

Residual scarring is an inevitable result of surgery. Some think that surgical scars will be invisible or hardly noticeable, or can be eradicated by further surgery. Sometimes scarring is minor or fades substantially with time, as is usually the case with eyelid surgery. With some procedures, scars can be hidden inside the ear, inside the nose, or in the hair line. Other procedures leave definite scars; the scars are a trade-off for the original defect that the surgery was intended to remove. For some patients, the distress caused by scarring may equal, if not surpass, distress over the original defect. Often it is merely substituting one blemish for another. Scarring can cancel out any psychological benefits achieved by correction of the perceived defect. A perfectionistic or narcissistic patient may pay inordinate attention to a scar and even come to see it as "mutilation." Even if patients are forewarned, they may not be fully prepared for the extent or appearance of the scarring. Unexpected results such as scarring can cause anger and bitterness, which is often directed at the surgeon. In order to avoid or lessen this reaction, the surgeon should explain in careful detail, what can be expected. Likewise, the patient needs to fully comprehend the extent to which scarring may occur.

Psychological Improvement After Surgery

Although improvement in appearance is one objective of cosmetic surgery, the overriding goal is emotional satisfaction and relief of distress about appearance. Some research has investigated whether patients indeed improve psychologically as the result of cosmetic surgery. In one early study, 70 percent of patients with a minimal deformity were assigned a psychiatric diagnosis, and half of them underwent cosmetic surgery. At follow-up six months later, 94 percent of those operated on showed a favorable psychological result.[23]

In one of the few controlled studies of psychological outcome after rhinoplasty, patients were compared to a group undergoing non-cosmetic surgery.[24] Both groups of patients were studied before surgery and twice afterwards, at 18 months and at 24 months. The study found the cosmetic surgery group tended to be somewhat agitated, tense, and depressed before surgery. Compared to the group receiving non-cosmetic surgery, the cosmetic surgery patients showed more psychological disturbance. Their agitation disappeared after surgery, and their energy and activity levels became more normal. After surgery, patients also seemed more self-confident in social situations and better able to establish, maintain, and enjoy relationships. They began to experiment with new clothes and hair styles, and their preoccupation with their perceived nose defects disappeared. The investigators concluded that while no major personality changes were noted after surgery, patients showed improvement in self-concept, a decrease in aggressive impulses, and less "somatization" (disturbed bodily functions with no apparent physical basis). These findings were confirmed in a later study also.[25]

In another study of rhinoplasty patients who were all under treatment by psychoanalysts, the therapists, rather than the patients, were interviewed.[26] Of 27 patients, 6 were deemed worse after surgery, 9 showed no psychological change, and 12 were improved. In many instances, the improvement came as a surprise to the therapist. (Interestingly, some therapists were not aware that a surgical change in the body could result in positive as well as negative effects.)

Research also has been done to ascertain psychological improvement following face-lift surgery.[27] At Johns Hopkins Hospital researchers reported 85 percent of face-lift patients experienced an improved sense of well-being. They had a greater sense of ease in social situations and were less self-critical after surgery. Most of the patients who were clearly depressed before the operation showed improvement in their depressive symptoms after surgery. About a quarter of the patients reported salary raises, awards, and new and better jobs, which they attributed to their enhanced appearance. About half described positive changes in their lives that included the formation of a new or better relationship or the termination of an old unsatisfactory relationship. (Some of the interviews done in this study took place as long as 12 years after surgery, and the findings may not be attributable to the operation.)

Another study reported that 52 percent of face-lift patients were judged by psychiatrists to show definite psychological improvement following surgery.[28] An increase in self-esteem and self-confidence was noted in 28 percent. As with the rhinoplasty patients after surgery, face-lift patients found themselves to be less anxious in social situations, more assertive, and more confident in their work. Patients who became worse after surgery tended to have midlife concerns that they had not revealed to their surgeons.

Goin and Goin label breast augmentation surgery "psychologically powerful and technically imperfect." Even when sponge implants were used in the 1950s, which inevitably turned hard and looked unnatural, most patients reported being "extremely pleased" with the results.[29] Self-image was enhanced, and patients gained self-confidence and lost self-consciousness. The prediction of psychiatrists in the 1950s that another fixation would develop —symptom substitution—did not come true.

Later, silicone gel implants replaced the sponges, though these too became the subject of controversy,[30] and saline-filled alternatives are now used in the United States. The vast majority of patients continued to confirm feeling better psychologically as the result of such surgery. One study of breast augmentation patients found that women felt more sexually desirable and more confident of their husbands' sexual interest, even though the husbands themselves reported feeling more or less neutral about the results of the surgery.[31] As these patients became more self-confident and less self-conscious their jealousy of other women diminished. Many reported feeling happy for the first time in their lives. Before surgery they often would not permit their breasts to be seen or touched; after surgery they were more likely to engage in "breast play," sometimes for the first time in their lives. They tended to have more interest in sex, and the frequency of intercourse increased. Some reported having orgasms for the first time in their lives. In spite of such improvements, most patients acknowledged that the surgery did not solve all problems. Jackie recounted her first sexual experience after surgery:

Jackie. Before surgery I used to hate being on top. I would look down at my sagging breasts, and I couldn't help but worry about what Tony must be thinking. For a long time before my surgery, I had a fantasy about what being on top would be like once I got my new breasts. I imagined I would feel really beautiful and powerful. When I finally got a chance to fulfill my fantasy after my surgery, it wasn't quite what I imagined, but it was good.

Patient Characteristics and Reactions to Cosmetic Surgery

In some instances small improvements or changes can result in great psychological improvement, but in other instances changes that seem strikingly good to others may not be experienced by the patient as positive and do not lead to psychological improvement. Those who are likely to be most happy with the results of cosmetic surgery are patients who are most bothered by self-consciousness, regardless of whether the perceived defect is minimal or marked. Similarly, people who are generally satisfied with their life and who have had a relatively stable childhood with positive regard from significant others are likely to make a good long-term adjustment. People who embrace a healthy lifestyle by eating well, by getting regular exercise, and by not smoking and drinking to excess are likely to do better than those who rely solely on cosmetic surgery to bring a transformation in appearance.

Research has tried to determine a link between various factors and post-operative complications. As yet no statistically significant relationship has been established between cosmetic surgery results and personality, motivation, severity of deficit, gender, or psychopathology.[32] The only clinically established contraindication to surgery is when there is psychosis with paranoid ideas about the body part to be operated on. Nevertheless, some warning signs of possible problems can be identified. These warning signs *may* signal an unfavorable reaction to cosmetic surgery.

Warning Signs

People are least likely to cope well with cosmetic surgery or might have an unfavorable psychological reaction if they:

- Have unrealistic expectations about what surgery can do.

- Are excessively concerned about a minimal defect.

- Are depressed prior to surgery.

- Are in a crisis (such as aging, divorce, retirement, widowhood) but don't recognize its relationship to the desire for surgery.

- Have a spouse or lover who strongly objects.

- Are seeking surgery primarily to please someone else.

- Want a total transformation.

- Are still grieving a loss.

- Need to be in control and deny their natural need to be cared for at times.

- Have a sudden urge for cosmetic surgery.

Summary

Patient satisfaction with the results of cosmetic surgery is uniformly high. Even so, patients may have to adjust to unexpected complications that can persist for some time or indefinitely, and they may have to come to terms with unmet expectations.

11

I Paid Good Money
for This?

Although his before-and-after rhinoplasty photographs showed dramatic improvement, the patient was very unhappy.[1] He complained that his nose looked like it belonged to someone else, that it looked "plastic." It was difficult for him to explain exactly what was wrong, but he could think of nothing else than how bad it looked. He was convinced that people stared at him in the street and were aware of his "nose job." Repeatedly he visited his surgeon, begging him to do something. "There is nothing to do," said the surgeon, "your nose looks great. Give it some time, you'll get used to it." One night the man appeared at an emergency room, having sliced off part of the tip of his nose with a razor.

In another case described by Dr. Marcia Goin, a woman in her mid-30s claimed that her "life was ruined" by eyelid surgery that had technically good results.[2] After the operation she became obsessive about her eyes and developed intense anxiety that interfered with her ability to work. She resigned from her high-level executive position and returned to her parents' home to live a reclusive life. At one point she spent some time in a psychiatric hospital. At various times she was diagnosed with depressive reaction, obsessive-compulsive personality, and borderline personality disorder.

In spite of objectively good results, some patients don't like how they look after surgery. They complain that all they got out of surgery was pain, scars, and a bill, they don't see much change in their appearance, or they don't like the changes they see. One study described nine women who had objectively good results after rhinoplasty but reported a loss of identity of their "old self."[3] All felt that "too much had been done." These women experienced difficulty integrating their altered appearance into their previous body image, making them unhappy with the results of the operation.

In rare instances dissatisfaction with results turns sinister. In 1977, a 45-year-old bachelor who had a nose reshaping to make himself more appealing was so upset when women continued to reject him that he reacted violently.[4] He broke into his surgeon's office and fired a pistol at the doctor and two nurses, killing all of them. Then he drove off wildly, eventually smashing the car and killing himself. An investigation showed he had made many attempts to talk with the doctor about his dissatisfaction with his nose, but the doctor's nurses had attempted to shield the doctor from what they thought was a demanding patient by not letting him see or talk to the doctor.

A similar tragedy was reported in *Allure* magazine.[5] In 1991, 60-year-old Beryl Challis murdered her surgeon, Dr. Selwyn Cohen, and then took her own life. She had obtained a face-lift from him, and although second opinions confirmed objectively good results, Challis complained of continuing and debilitating pain. She wanted Dr. Cohen to do more surgery to find and correct the source of pain. When he refused, she took desperate action.

Challis's face-lift was not her first cosmetic surgery operation. She first consulted Dr. Cohen in 1987 requesting a second rhinoplasty to refine surgery provided by another surgeon. The next year she returned for liposuction of the abdomen and thighs. Not satisfied, she asked for additional liposuction. In addition to being an insatiable surgery patient, she was notable for her secrecy (she insisted that her husband not know about her surgeries) and for her need of attention from the doctor and his staff. She created reasons to visit the doctor and sometimes would just come and sit in the office with no appointment. In the 12 months before her death, she had more than 30 office visits with Dr. Cohen in addition to her casual visits. Dr. Cohen did his best to respond to this patient's complaints and needs. Although he eventually referred her to a psychiatrist, she did not keep any of several psychiatric appointments. In a suicide letter to Dr. Cohen she complained about her hair loss and itching scalp, the length of her incision, the extent of her brow-lift, the tightness of her muscles, her 11 months of "excruciating pain," and her anger at him for refusing her further surgery.

The Doctor/Patient Relationship

Although the majority who undergo cosmetic surgery are pleased with their results, according to one study 49 percent of plastic surgeons are sued at least once in their careers by a disgruntled patient.[6] In only a small percent of these cases is the patient displeased with the *results* of the surgery. The most frequent reason for lawsuits is lack of rapport between surgeon and patient.

Objectively bad results, surgeon negligence, or complications from surgery accounted for only about a fourth of lawsuits. In the list Why Patients Sue, the importance of non-surgery factors is clear. Most of the time what prompts patient dissatisfaction leading to a lawsuit is a problem in the doctor/patient relationship.

Why Patients Sue

Reasons	Percent of Lawsuits
Lack of rapport between surgeon and patient	51.6
Unrealistic patient expectations	17.0
Poor surgical results	14.5
Poor selection of patients	6.5
Surgeon negligence	4.8
Post-operative complications	4.0
Surgeon's insensitivity to patient's emotional needs	1.6

Wright, M. R. (1986). Surgical addiction: A complication of modern surgery? *Archives of Otolaryngology and Head and Neck Surgery, 112,* 870-872.

Marjorie complained that when she came out of the anesthesia, her surgeon and the nurses were gone. Only the anesthesiologist had bothered to stay with her. She explained that she felt alone and abandoned. Later, she complained to her surgeon that parts of her face didn't seem quite right, but he appeared annoyed by her complaints. She called his office repeatedly to ask that something be done, but the office nurse said he was too busy to come to the phone. Marjorie filed a lawsuit for nerve damage behind her ear.

Research shows that surgeons and their staff may not always provide the emotional support a patient needs. Nurses who attend cosmetic surgery patients sometimes have difficulty being sympathetic.[7] They may become irritated with demands that take up time and energy that may seem better spent with "legitimately" sick patients. (One source of such irritation can be the social taboos about cosmetic surgery, discussed in Chapter 9.) Plastic surgeons themselves may fail to offer psychological help when needed.[8] They may be uncomfortable with emotional problems, and dealing with emotional issues is not part of their training. It is not in their nature or in their daily routine to probe for psychological pain. Often they are so busy it doesn't occur to them to check for this. Finally, surgeons may lack confidence in dealing with such issues.

Leanne, whose experience with a hematoma was described in Chapter 7, was refused pain medication by her doctor, who said he didn't believe in it. Although this was upsetting to her, the doctor's failure to notice her emotional needs was even more upsetting. After the surgeon drained the hematoma that developed nine days after surgery, he gave her the name of another doctor to call in case there were any further complications. He explained that he was going on vacation and wouldn't be available. Leanne understood that doctors take vacations, but was frightened that something else might happen while he was gone. Putting herself in the hands of a strange doctor merely added to her stress. In fact, her recovery proceeded without incident. Still, Leanne was upset that even after returning from vacation he did not contact her again to see how she was doing. "I'd never go to him again," she declared. "I won't recommend him to anyone."

Patients often don't ask for emotional support from their surgeons, either because they are too shy or they feel they have no right to bother the doctor about such matters. Usually, they see the doctor's role as being concerned with physical, not emotional health, and they don't want to displease the surgeon by bringing up emotional issues. Nevertheless, patients often need emotional support. They need to be prepared to solicit it, if not from the plastic surgeon and his staff, then from a therapist trained to provide it.

Psychiatric Disturbance and Cosmetic Surgery

In some cases a person with a preexisting psychiatric impairment seeks cosmetic surgery, and there is a danger that surgery can trigger an exacerbation of this underlying disturbance. Perhaps because rhinoplasty is a type-changing operation, it is associated far more frequently with post-operative psychiatric disturbance than other cosmetic procedures. One case report described a Caucasian woman who complained that her rhinoplasty made her look negroid.[9] It was later revealed that she had had a long-standing psychotic delusion that her father (whom she had never seen) was black, and the surgery became part of this delusion. In yet another case, the plastic surgeon was unaware that a schizophrenic patient was convinced that bad odors emanated from her nose. When she complained that the rhinoplasty operation had not helped, the surgeon refused to operate again contending that the operation had an objectively good result. The patient later attempted suicide. Psychotic delusions are frequently associated with schizophrenia, and cosmetic surgery can exacerbate the patient's psychosis.[10]

Although anxiety and depressive symptoms occur quite frequently after a face-lift, serious psychotic decompensation (the breakdown of ability to cope with the demands of life) is surprisingly uncommon. Because a face-lift is viewed as a primarily restorative, rather than type-changing operation, it is not usually associated with significant psychiatric disturbance. A face-lift can impact body image, especially in the early post-operative period, because of the temporary but significant physical changes—bruising, swelling, and numbness. Nevertheless, a case has been reported in which a face-lift was aesthetically satisfactory, but the patient had an unusually severe psychological response:[11]

> *Carey.* Carey was a 45-year-old divorced white female who complained of jowling and excessive skin. She wanted her youthful appearance restored. Carey appeared younger than her stated age and had had two previous operations, one for correction of torticollis (wryneck) at age 16 and eyelid surgery three years before the current surgery. Both were without complications. The patient was polite and cooperative with no indications of abnormal behavior or mood. She was given the usual pain medication. Approximately 24 hours after the operation and shortly before discharge, there was a dramatic change in the patient's behavior. She become anxious and visibly upset, complaining bitterly of "pain and terrible swelling" in her face. Carey became increasingly paranoid, and her mood fluctuated between cheerful optimism and angry and tearful pessimism. Her erratic and unstable behavior and emotional state persisted for five weeks, gradually resolving. A mild depression emerged and persisted for three months. Gradually she accepted her surgical result and finally expressed satisfaction about six months later. In addition to a borderline personality disorder, this patient had had a lifelong preoccupation with her appearance and an unshakable belief in her own ugliness. This body image disturbance made her vulnerable to psychotic breakdown.

In some cases, surgery itself can induce a psychiatric disturbance. As discussed earlier in Chapter 7 with regard to rhinoplasties, sometimes this is the result of events that occur during the operation itself, particularly if a local anesthesia is used. John and Marcia Goin were the first to assert that sometimes severe and potentially serious emotional reactions begin during an operation done under a local anesthesia.[12] Often the surgeon and his staff are unaware of this problem. The Goins give several examples of what can happen during an operation to cause psychological problems.

In one case, the wife of another physician had a face-lift under local anesthesia. Although prior to the operation she seemed like a "routine patient" and presented no evidence of disturbance, the day following the operation she was surly and withdrawn. Later, she gave her psychiatrist a detailed account of a severe paranoid delusion that began during her operation. Because of a conversation between the surgeon and his staff that she was able to overhear during the operation, she concluded that the surgeon was "on edge" and touchy. As the operation progressed she became more and more frightened that something would go wrong if the surgeon became further upset. At one point she felt pain, and she couldn't stop herself from crying out. At this point the surgeon became very quiet (actually, he paused to inject additional anesthetic), and she thought he did this to cover his anger at her for complaining. When the surgeon commented that he would let her rest for a moment she interpreted this as a threat that if she complained again he would terminate the operation while half-finished. She remained quiet and tried to be a "good patient," but one in sheer terror.

The day after the operation she lay immobile, convinced that any movement would undo the operation, which she believed the surgeon in his anger had done in a purposefully superficial manner so that it would fall apart if she moved. Finally, several days later, she was able to speak rationally about these irrational thoughts. The Goins point out the parallel between the patient's response to the surgeon and her unexpressed feelings about her own physician-husband, toward whom she felt great anger and had serious doubts about his treatment of her in their marriage. Six months later, vestiges of her paranoid reaction remained. She complained that one side of her face was pulled too tight and believed this was a deliberate act of retaliation by the surgeon for her complaint of pain during the operation.

In another case reported by the Goins, a woman overheard conversation between the surgeon and his nurse that led to the conviction her real surgeon was absent and an imposter was operating on her. Three weeks after the operation, she admitted to "going a little crazy" during the operation, and her paranoia resolved. As the Goins explain, local anesthesia reduces or alters normal sensory input which, together with the emotional stress induced by surgery, makes patients especially vulnerable to misinterpretations of overheard conversations.

Cases of Bad Results

Sometimes the results of cosmetic surgery are objectively bad. Testimony given before the Congressional Subcommittee on Regulation, Business Opportunities, and Energy in 1989 provides some insight into just how wrong things can go.[13] Joyce P., a cosmetic surgery patient, gave a statement to the congressional investigation of the cosmetic surgery business.[14] She had made what appeared to be a thorough verification of the credentials of the surgeon she wanted to use. She called the American Medical Association and was told the doctor was a "member in good standing." She learned later that meant he had paid his dues. She had called the California Board of Medical Quality Assurance and was told they had "nothing on him." She learned later that in fact 11 lawsuits had been filed against him, but because he had not been proven guilty in any of the cases, the board couldn't reveal the fact of these complaints. (Out-of-court settlements avoid the verdict of "guilty.") Joyce also noted that the surgeon was board certified by the Board of Cosmetic Surgeons. She was not aware that that is a self-designated board not recognized by the American Board of Medical Specialties (ABMS). (A list of boards recognized by the ABMS is given in the appendix along with a list of self-designated boards which are not recognized by the ABMS.) She checked with the University of California at Davis, which the surgeon listed as a source of his education, and was told he may have attended a seminar there. She asked for the names of former patients and talked with three of them. Because of his impressive credentials and by talking with his former patients, she thought she had reason to believe this surgeon was a good choice.

In 1984 Joyce allowed this surgeon to perform a tummy tuck operation. Nine days later, problems began to appear. Fluid began to seep from the wound through the bandage; parts of the wound area had turned black and another part was red, bloody, and pussy. The doctor confirmed that an infection had set in and prescribed antibiotics. He assured her it would be "okay." Nevertheless, it worsened. The wound began to have a terrible odor, and Joyce was coughing, becoming short of breath, and getting weaker. Despite repeated visits to the surgeon and changes in treatment, she continued to worsen. Against the advice of her first surgeon she sought a second opinion from another doctor. The second doctor immediately sent her to the emergency room, and because of the quick work of a team of specialists and the support of a hospital Joyce's life was saved. Repeated hospitalizations were necessary even after the initial emergency intervention. As a result of these medical problems Joyce lost her health and her business. Still, she counts herself as lucky. Two months after Joyce's tummy tuck surgery, the same doctor performed this operation on a 36 year-old nurse. Infection set in, and she died. In 1987 the doctor's license to practice was finally revoked. Patients can die from the medical malpractice of surgeons not qualified to do a particular plastic surgery operation.

In another case, Angela B. was careful to choose a board certified plastic surgeon for her liposuction to remove saddlebags from her legs. The operation was supposed to take 45 minutes but lasted two hours because the lipo machine kept breaking down. The nurse remarked that she felt the doctor had removed "lots more fat than I thought you had." Initially Angela felt fine, but about three or four weeks after the surgery she noticed her right thigh was developing a large cavity and was sensitive to touch. When she saw her surgeon, he acknowledged that too much fat had been removed. He said that a fat graft (injection of fat from other parts of the body into the area where additional fat is desired) might be necessary to correct the problem, but advised that the cavity would probably fill in by itself. Angela's leg continued to get worse. The cavity widened to six inches long and six inches wide, running down the front of her right thigh. "I could place my whole hand in the area. I could feel the muscle and the bone in my leg. The area was rock-hard and it hurt." Then her knee began to swell and she could not bend her leg nor put pressure on it. Again she returned to her doctor, who assured her, "Don't worry. Scar tissue is making the leg hard. Gradually the knee will return to normal. It's swollen due to the pressure of the scar tissue in your leg."

After months of repeat visits without getting any relief, Angela sought opinions from several other surgeons. Eventually she found one who had extensive experience performing liposurgery. He took a long time talking with her, measuring her leg, taking pictures, and planning the fat graft that would correct the problem. The doctor wrote prescriptions in advance for the antibiotics and pain pills that Angela would need when she returned home after the operation. She reported that unlike the other doctors she consulted this doctor made her feel comfortable and safe. "He practiced careful medicine, taking blood tests and being scrupulously careful about sterile instruments and the dangers of infection." After the sedation took effect, the surgeon removed fat from her stomach and upper arms to fill in the cavity in her right leg. "Afterwards my right leg was severely swollen and hurt with a throbbing intensity." It would take three weeks before she would know if the fat graft had taken. "I realized then that undergoing surgery to become slim and trim was not an issue to be considered trivially. Liposuction is surgery. Things can and do go wrong."

An article in *Reader's Digest* reported the experience of Elaine.[15] To heighten her cheekbones she had silicone injections in her cheeks every 3 weeks for 18 months. For a while she looked lovely. Then the silicone grew granite-hard, and chunks of it began shifting. Her once beautiful face became distorted and gargoyle-like. Elaine went from doctor to doctor until she finally found a surgeon who thought he could correct the problem. After enduring numerous other operations at great cost, the shape of her face is back to normal, but her skin is discolored a reddish blue—the unerasable aftermath of silicone injections.

Most surgeons are willing to do additional operations if necessary to correct complications or bad results. (Doctors may decline to do additional surgery if they feel the results are acceptable and the patient's response is not well founded.) Patients may not accept an offer of additional surgery. It is often a sensitive issue, and if the undesirable results can be hidden, as in breast surgery, the patient may decide to put it out of her mind. One woman who had an unsuccessful breast reduction spoke of her attempt not to think about it and endure discomfort as the scar tissue chafed against her bra. Ann refused further surgical intervention:

> *Ann.* Ann had long thought of herself as an unattractive woman who lacked anything a man would want. She was convinced that men were interested only in women with big breasts. After several years of deliberation, she decided to have a breast augmentation. Several weeks after an uneventful operation, Ann developed a wound infection in her left breast that resulted in sloughing of tissue and the ultimate removal of the implant on that side. To her horror, her breasts were now asymmetrical and disfigured, adding one more aspect to her longstanding self-dislike. Although the doctor was willing to try again and indicated there was a good

chance of a satisfactory result, Ann refused. She became depressed and was unable to return to work. She eventually improved emotionally but continued to have great difficulty functioning socially. Ann continues to obsess about suing the surgeon for having "mutilated" her, but she has not taken action.

What Causes Bad Results?

Many things can go wrong and cause bad results. In rare instances equipment may fail, as in the case of Angela B. Bad results have been attributed to disputed products such as silicone gel breast implants or to the inappropriate use of products. Most often, tragedy can be attributed to inexperienced, untrained, or inadequately trained doctors who try to do plastic surgery. The previously mentioned *Reader's Digest* article describes other cases of bad results by unscrupulous, unskilled practitioners with little or no formal training.[16] The need to carefully assess a doctor's qualifications is detailed in Chapter 6. Unfortunately, it is perfectly legal for anyone with an M.D. degree to perform any medical procedure. The only protection the consumer has is to carefully assess the doctor's qualifications and proceed cautiously.

Summary

A number of factors contribute to patient dissatisfaction with objectively good results. In some cases, patients seek cosmetic surgery for the wrong reasons, or they have unrealistic expectations of what surgery will do for them. Patients who seek surgery to please someone else or who do it impulsively may not be satisfied. In other cases, patients have difficulty integrating changes with their body image. When patients fail to bring concerns or complaints to a surgeon's attention, they may end up complaining about objectively good results. A few patients have preexisting psychological problems that are not helped or may be exacerbated by cosmetic surgery.

Sometimes patient dissatisfaction with results is attributable to the surgeon.[17] When surgeons or their staff fail to respond to patients' emotional needs or to listen empathetically to problems or complaints, the doctor/patient relationship is likely to be impaired and lead to patient dissatisfaction. The surgeon may fail to prepare the patient fully about what to expect during and after the procedure, or he may minimize what is involved. Sometimes the surgeon fails to adequately interview and carefully evaluate a prospective patient or have the patient evaluated by a therapist if indicated. Although psychiatric impairment is not, in and of itself, a necessary disqualifier for cosmetic surgery, care must be taken that surgery is not likely to exacerbate a preexisting condition. Tragic results occur most frequently when the doctor performing the operation is untrained or unqualified. An important warning is, "Buyer beware."

12

Surgery or Therapy?

When Susan initially sought therapy for reasons unrelated to cosmetic surgery she was in a crisis. At age 37, she had a secret crush on a man who was a distant friend and had frequently fantasized about having a relationship with him. When she learned that he was about to marry someone else she was devastated. Susan had always been shy and apprehensive around people and had never had many friends, let alone a love relationship. Her life consisted of working five days a week as a bookkeeper and a solitary hobby that required no other person's participation. Through the encouragement and support of her therapist, Susan gradually began to overcome her fear of criticism and rejection by others and to extend herself to make new friends. Despite progress in taking more interpersonal risks, Susan encountered yet another crisis about ten months into therapy. She was diagnosed with breast cancer. At first she was so traumatized that she refused to return to the doctor to discuss further treatment, but with emotional support from her therapist she eventually underwent a mastectomy of her right breast. This was followed by reconstruction of the right breast and augmentation of the remaining breast. This turned out to be an important turning point for Susan. Her self-confidence increased dramatically, and she became more outgoing. She developed a real relationship with a man and, at last contact, reported being "happier than I've ever been in my life."

Was it therapy that helped Susan overcome her need to avoid others in order to protect herself from possible criticism? Was it facing down the threat of cancer and the physical mutilation that this disease can bring? Even though her breasts had not been discussed as a source of self-consciousness prior to the cancer diagnosis, did Susan actually have a body image problem that the plastic surgery alleviated? Most likely the therapy provided a crucial sense of increased self-efficacy, and the surgery contributed to an improved body image, both of which allowed Susan to create more positive and satisfactory relationships. Susan's experience indicates that therapy and surgery can complement each other.

Anita, whose story was told in Chapter 9, was also in therapy when she decided to go ahead with breast augmentation surgery. Her therapist, advised against it. "You'll regret it," he predicted. Anita decided that as a male he could not understand her motivation, and she also was having difficulty connecting with him as her therapist. She ignored his prediction and went ahead with surgery. Later, with a different therapist Anita began to explore and understand the dynamics of her two surgeries and her ultimate disillusionment:

> *Anita.* I understand now how being an adopted child had a lot to do with my experience. I had the good fortune to be adopted by a wealthy family, and I've always supposed that my real parents aren't so fortunate. In that sense, I felt like a fraud even before I got my boobs done. All the advantages and trappings of a comfortable life weren't really mine. After my surgery, I couldn't bring myself to tell my family. They must have wondered what was going on with me—first I had no boobs, then I had big boobs, now I have no boobs. I realize now that at age 26, when I got my first set of implants, I really had not developed a firm sense of self. I thought I wanted to look sexy and attract lots of attention, and I did. But I also had this nagging feeling of being a fraud. It's only now, at age 35, that I really feel I know myself. I'm getting married soon, and my husband-to-be knew me before when I had big boobs. He told me, "Honey, I don't care what you have in your bra. I care about you." That's now true for me too. I don't feel like a fraud any more. My therapy helped me work through my issues about being adopted and become more self-accepting as well. It's just too bad that I had to end up with lots of scars before I got to this point.

Both Susan and Anita were in therapy at the time they had cosmetic surgery. In Susan's case the therapy and the cosmetic surgery worked synergistically to promote better social functioning and psychological improvement. Although Anita talked with her first therapist about her intention to get breast augmentation, she didn't see her therapist's concern as particularly relevant. Anita's second course of therapy helped her work through issues that existed before her cosmetic surgery and helped her accept the choices she had made. She eventually decided to have her breast augmentation reversed.

Those seeking cosmetic surgery usually regard themselves as psychologically healthy. They do not regard wanting cosmetic surgery as indicative of psychological dysfunction, but rather as a way of coping actively with their lives. Surgery is regarded as a logical cure for a perceived defect in appearance, the alteration of which is expected to reduce self-consciousness, increase self-confidence and self-esteem, and generally provide a feeling of improved well-being. Nevertheless, there are times when therapy may be a better solution than surgery. If Anita had been willing to work through some painful issues initially, she probably would not have had breast augmentation. Often cosmetic surgery is perceived as quicker and easier than psychotherapy. Surgery requires less activity on the part of the patient and is often seen as less time consuming and possibly less costly than psychotherapy.

Referral to a Therapist

Sometimes plastic surgeons refer prospective patients to a therapist for consultation.[1] Most people who seek cosmetic surgery strongly resent being asked to go for a psychiatric consultation, which they interpret as an insinuation that they have psychological problems or conflicts. If there are problems, a prospective patient usually considers them to be caused by the cosmetic defect or unrelated to it. When surgeons suggest a patient see a therapist for consultation, the patient may not follow through. Beryl Challis, mentioned in Chapter 11, was referred several times by her surgeon, Dr. Cohen, who felt she should see a psychiatrist for a consultation. Challis made several appointments but did not keep them. In hindsight, therapy, rather than surgery, would have been a better choice for her.

Reasons for a Referral

Referring a patient for a psychiatric consultation does not necessarily mean the surgeon thinks the patient has a psychological conflict or abnormality. Usually when a surgeon refers a patient to a psychotherapist it is not to determine how psychologically disturbed a patient is, but to assess how well this patient is likely to cope with cosmetic surgery. A psychiatric consultation may be recommended for a number of different reasons. The surgeon may want the psychotherapist to assess the emotional suitability of the patient for surgery. Time is often limited in the consultation between the surgeon and a prospective patient, and the surgeon may not feel able to do the kind of assessment needed, particularly if the patient appears to be in some kind of crisis or emotional turmoil. The psychotherapist can take more time and is more experienced in exploring the prospective patient's relationships and coping patterns and in dealing with partners and whole families.

The important question the surgeon needs to have answered is, Will my patient be made worse psychologically by the proposed operation? If the surgeon suspects that a prospective patient is in the midst of a life crisis and is seeking surgery as a means of coping, the surgeon may want the input of a therapist. (Of course, a therapist with a bias against cosmetic surgery should be avoided.) A consultation can help decide whether to proceed with cosmetic surgery or whether therapy is more appropriate. Perhaps the patient would benefit from body image therapy before cosmetic surgery. Sometimes the surgeon wants a patient to establish rapport with a psychotherapist in advance of surgery so that the therapist can be available for support and treatment during the post-operative period if necessary. Occasionally, patients experience a difficult transition (for example, the ugly duckling-to-swan problem) and benefit from the support of a psychotherapist. A surgeon may refer a prospective patient to a psychotherapist because he feels uneasy about a patient or because he finds the patient difficult or trying. In this case, it is the surgeon who needs the psychotherapist's guidance in how to serve the needs of his patient.

People seeking cosmetic surgery range from stable individuals with a strong sense of self to the emotionally fragile or frankly psychotic. Fragile or psychotic people need to be carefully evaluated and given appropriate therapeutic support if the decision is made to proceed with surgery. Under the right conditions psychiatrically impaired patients may be helped by cosmetic surgery, and the support and guidance of a psychotherapist can be crucial. The psychotherapist is an important part of a team that includes the patient, the surgeon, and other medical professionals who have the best interests of the patient at heart.

What the Therapist Needs to Know

When a prospective cosmetic surgery patient sees a psychotherapist at a surgeon's request, the therapist needs to explore a variety of issues. The therapist will want to know how long the patient has been unhappy with the body part to be altered and its emotional significance to this patient. A key question is, Why now? What is prompting cosmetic surgery at this time? Is the patient in a life crisis? If so, is the request for the operation a positive, adaptive step or an attempt to deny the underlying problem? (Being in a crisis is not always a counterindication to surgery.) Are family and friends generally supportive or hostile to the proposed operation? Who is the patient planning to tell, and why or why not? Does the patient expect any negative reactions, and how would she handle them? Is the patient's primary motivation for surgery to improve her self-image or self-esteem, or to please or influence someone else? Motives that involve a hoped-for effect on someone else are often unrealizable and unrealistic.

Benefits of a Referral

When a prospective cosmetic surgery patient sees a psychotherapist for consultation he or she is getting a second professional's perspective and as-

sistance to ensure the best possible results. Seeking the advice of a psychotherapist is especially important if the patient is ambivalent about cosmetic
surgery, if the patient feels pressured by others, or if the surgery is perceived
as a solution to a larger life problem. Ultimately, the determining factor for a
good outcome of cosmetic surgery is the patient's ability to cope. A psychotherapist can often help the patient plan and adapt to the challenges cosmetic
surgery can present.

Coping Skills

The ability to conceive of a "possible self" and the desire to have cosmetic
surgery is not usually a sign of pathology. Rather, it is often a creative act of
adaptation in response to a psychologically stressful situation—coping with
the self-consciousness and distress associated with a perceived defect in appearance.[2] The real issue in deciding whether surgery or therapy is more appropriate has to do with the coping skills and resources the patient brings to
each stage of the process. Not only will the patient have to cope with the
physical and emotional trauma that is frequently present in the early stages
of recovery, he or she will be challenged to cope at each step of the way, from
perceiving a deficit in appearance to deciding whether to proceed with surgery, from preparing for surgery to managing the later stages of recovery.

Initiating the process of obtaining cosmetic surgery is only the first in a
series of challenges. In the consultation with a surgeon the patient must cope
with the often alarming information about risks associated with cosmetic surgery. Preparing for the operation can involve a variety of coping efforts such
as losing weight or quitting smoking. During the early recovery period the
patient must cope with inevitable pain and physical trauma. Coping is required to deal with unexpected complications and unmet expectations. Not
only is "coping" a reasonable explanation for seeking surgery it also helps
explain outcome and the degree of ease or difficulty patients have in recovery.
Patients with poor coping skills are likely to have a harder time than those
with good ones.

A Coping Model

Arthur A. Stone, Ph.D., of the State University of New York and his
colleague Laura S. Porter, M.A., posit a way of understanding the relationship
between psychological coping and medical problems.[3] Coping refers to the
constantly changing thoughts and actions used to manage situations that are
difficult or threatening, either to physical or emotional health. Stone and Porter's definition is based on a theory originated by Richard Lazarus known as
the transactional model of stress and coping.[4] The model consists of three
stages: the occurrence of an event, the appraisal process, and the coping effort.

The first stage in coping with stress is the occurrence of an event or
problem. An event may develop quickly, as in discovering a lump in the

breast, or it may develop over time, as in increasing self-consciousness about a large nose. Many different kinds of events or problems elicit coping efforts related to cosmetic surgery, such as experiencing a perceived defect in appearance, anticipating a painful or dangerous procedure, making a commitment to obtain cosmetic surgery, actually having surgery, or recognizing that one must live with unanticipated complications.

The next stage of the transactional model is the appraisal of the event or problem—how threatening to physical or emotional health is it? This involves judgments about the severity, degree of threat, and controllability of the problem. Appraisal is influenced by both situational and individual factors and is critical in determining what coping strategies are chosen. In finding a lump in the breast, the event would probably be judged as relatively uncontrollable and extremely threatening. Becoming increasingly distressed over a large nose is likely to be seen as more controllable (cosmetic surgery could modify it) if a person has the resources and social support necessary to obtain cosmetic surgery.

Situations differ in how controllable they seem to be. For those who see cosmetic surgery as an available option, an unsightly nose is relatively controllable. Those who reject cosmetic surgery may have no other solution than to learn to live with their deficit. People also differ in the amount of control they feel they need and have. Someone who perceives herself to have a high level of control is more likely to seek a consultation with a plastic surgeon than one who has a low sense of control, for example, someone who knows her spouse will oppose her desire to change her nose. Those who need to feel in control but are not are more vulnerable to developing depression especially during recovery from surgery. It is important to note that the appraisal stage is dynamic and changing. As the problem is assessed over time, how threatening it is and what should be done about it are repeatedly reevaluated. At some point, a previously low-level threat can reach a higher level and trigger efforts to cope. Initiating efforts to cope is the third stage of the transactional model.

Coping Strategies

Research into coping is still in its infancy and has focused primarily on cancer patients.[5] Much of what has been learned can be applied to cosmetic surgery as well. The decision to undergo cosmetic surgery and recovery are sources of stress that require coping. People attempt to cope with stress in many ways, both consciously and unconsciously. Access to adequate social support is an important coping resource, and seeking emotional support or advice of others is generally considered to be a good, or adaptive, strategy. Another coping strategy is distancing oneself from the problem. This may be done consciously by purposefully ignoring information about a problem or unconsciously by "forgetting" the information. The distancing strategy, also known as denial, is generally thought to be nonadaptive.

Whether a particular strategy is adaptive or not depends on the situation. Those who rely mainly on the advice of others or are passive about their needs and their desire for cosmetic surgery exhibit nonadaptive coping. However, the ability to accept emotional support from others, especially in the early stages of recovery, is an adaptive coping strategy. The ability to distance oneself from pain in the early recovery stages can be adaptive, but distancing oneself from information about risks at the decision stage is not adaptive.

Two other ways of coping involve the kind of attention a person pays to threat.[6] When threatened, some people seek more information and pay close attention to threat cues. These people are called *monitors*. Those who avoid or distract themselves from threat-relevant information are known as *blunters*. Monitors have a hypervigilant style and often experience anxiety and distress in the face of threat. Because of their vigilance and concern they often suffer intrusive thoughts about a threat and exaggerate the level of actual risk by overfocusing on the problem. A monitor who seeks a consultation about cosmetic surgery may become overly frightened by the surgeon's discussion of risks and decide against proceeding further or may cancel surgery after initially scheduling it. If somehow the monitor is able to proceed with the operation, she may focus intensively on the pain and physical trauma that inevitably accompanies surgery and become increasingly distressed and anxious. Although monitors are vulnerable to anxiety and distress in the face of a threatening event, they tend to follow the doctor's orders and adhere to recommended health regimens.

In contrast to monitors, blunters prefer less information. Blunters employ the denial or distancing strategy. They avoid information that raises anxiety by either not attending to it, or by forgetting it, or by distracting themselves and focusing attention elsewhere. Blunters may be advised of risks and possible complications prior to surgery, but they are not affected by this information because they are able to deny or suppress the information and focus selectively on the expected benefits of the operation.

A psychiatric consultation or a brief course of therapy can be very helpful to monitors. The goal is to help them accurately assess risk information and reduce exaggerated perceptions of risk, minimizing intrusive thoughts and psychological distress without compromising their ability to adhere to medical advice.[7] Blunters also need assistance in learning to tolerate and manage anxiety so they can integrate information on risk and make better decisions. Often blunters need to feel in control, and they use the denial strategy to manage relatively uncontrollable threats. Another goal of therapy with blunters is to help them understand their need for control as a means of managing anxiety and develop greater tolerance for uncertainty.

How controllable a problem is perceived to be affects the kind of coping efforts used. If an event is seen as controllable, a person will alter conditions by taking action. This is called *problem-focused coping*. If a problem seems less controllable (enduring long-term discomfort or pain, for example), coping attempts are likely to focus on accepting and adjusting to the condition. This is called *emotion-focused coping*, which is an internal strategy of revising beliefs, attitudes, and thoughts about the stressor.

Coping efforts fail when the wrong strategy is used. Beryl Challis demanded more surgery, a problem-focused coping strategy, to alleviate the pain she experienced after cosmetic surgery. A more appropriate strategy would have been to learn to cope with the pain through distraction, guided imagery, meditation, or another emotion-focused coping strategy. Had Challis kept any of the appointments she made with a therapist, she might have been helped to cope more effectively. When a person does not cope adequately the outcome is likely to be depression rather than a satisfactory adjustment.

Coping and Illness

A considerable amount of research suggests that the mind affects the body. Mood, emotion, and thought influence the body's ability to resist or recover from illness. Negativity may adversely affect immunity and the endocrine and nervous systems. Sometimes the body expresses by illness what is unable to be faced psychologically.[8] How threatening and controllable an event is and the coping efforts used are likely to generate some kind of emotional response. Maintaining a positive attitude about a problem and having the support of important others aids the selection of appropriate strategies to cope with stress. Poor coping can interfere with taking appropriate action in a timely fashion, seeking help from others, perceiving of symptoms, or experiencing a sense of well-being.

Coping and the Doctor/Patient Relationship

Inadequate coping efforts can disrupt effective communication between doctor and patient. The patient who tries to cope with unexpected complications by distancing herself from the doctor or additional medical procedures may put herself at risk. Patients who fail to inform their doctors that they don't comprehend the information given or don't ask questions or express feelings are using a distancing strategy for coping with anxiety. An anxious and hypervigilant patient may try the doctor's patience, setting the stage for a deterioration of the doctor/patient relationship. Coping efforts can have direct effects on the doctor/patient relationship as well as on emotions. Coping affects health and well-being.

Good Coping Skills

Coping skills specific to medical procedures are still under study, but much is known about what constitutes good coping skills in general. The ability to think and act positively facilitates coping. Positive coping behaviors are the ability to express feelings and emotions appropriately, manage conflict and negative emotions, create positive relationships, and create, maintain, and access adequate social support. Good self-care practices are important— healthy eating, regular exercise, good hygiene, and regular medical care. Thinking skills facilitate good coping and begin with setting reachable goals and creating realistic expectations. Positive thinking means being adaptive and flexible. There is a high ratio of positive to negative self-talk and an ability to maintain a positive outlook without ignoring negative or threat-relevant information. Psychotherapy can be helpful in developing good coping skills.

Choosing a Therapist

Finding the right therapist can be challenging but referrals are available from a variety of sources. Physicians, other therapists, mental health practitioners, nurses, religious leaders, and school or job counselors are all good leads for getting the name of a potential therapist. It may also be helpful to ask for a referral from a friend or relative whose contact is not personal, that is, they do not have a current therapeutic relationship with that therapist.

Clearly, an important factor in choosing a therapist is to be sure he or she has expertise in body image issues and does not hold a particular bias against cosmetic surgery. Asking therapists about their experience and training in these areas, and whether they have a particular bias is perfectly appropriate. Often it is possible to get a referral to a qualified psychotherapist from a plastic surgeon. It is preferable to get two or three names from the surgeon and ask how the recommended therapists differ from each other.

Therapists have different kinds of training for various academic or professional degrees. Psychiatry is the medical specialty that seeks to study, diagnose, and treat mental illness. A psychiatrist holds a degree (generally an M.D.) from a medical school and usually has completed a three- or four-year residency focusing on mental health and mental illness problems. As physicians, psychiatrists are uniquely qualified to prescribe psychotropic medications such as anti-depressants and anti-psychotics. Usually they have completed a psychiatric residency, though not all physicians who practice psychiatry have necessarily undergone any special training or passed the medical specialty board in psychiatry. In the United States, any physician licensed to practice medicine may hang out a shingle stating he practices psychiatry. Generally, board certified psychiatrists are more likely to possess the greatest knowledge in the field.

Psychologists providing mental health services may hold either a Ph.D. or a Psy.D. degree. In addition to completing a formal internship they receive training in one or more therapeutic orientations, such as psychodynamic, cognitive, behavioral, family systems, humanistic, and so on. The Ph.D. indicates expertise and training in research; the Psy.D. emphasizes clinical work. Some Ph.D. psychologists primarily do research, while others may earn their living as clinical psychologists or counseling psychologists. Special training in testing and assessment distinguishes psychologists from other mental health professionals. Currently, psychologists cannot prescribe medications.

Psychotherapists may hold degrees other than the M.D., Ph.D., or Psy.D. Psychotherapy is also provided by licensed clinical social workers (L.C.S.W.s); marriage, family, and child counselors (M.F.C.C.s), and master's level practitioners (M.A.s). These professionals may not have as much academic training as Ph.D.s, but they complete a comparable number of training hours in preparation for licensing. Other mental health professionals who may provide therapy include psychiatric social workers, psychiatric nurses, pastoral counselors, and unlicensed therapists in supervised training.

Aside from the therapist's credentials, experience, and training, the most important consideration in choosing a therapist is the client's own reactions to the therapist. Feeling safe, understood, and comfortable with a particular therapist is most important.

Summary

People seeking cosmetic surgery are generally psychologically healthy, but there are times when a psychiatric consultation is useful. Occasionally, therapy rather than surgery is indicated. When a cosmetic surgery patient is referred for psychiatric evaluation, the key question is not how psychologically impaired she is but how well will she cope with surgery and will she improve as a result? Psychopathology, in and of itself, is not a sufficient reason to refuse cosmetic surgery to a patient. There are cases in which a patient is significantly impaired psychologically, but cosmetic surgery does not interfere and even improves the patient's situation to some extent. Furthermore, research has found that cosmetic surgery can produce a definite improvement in those with moderate to mild psychopathology. It appears that surgery itself can be a form of psychotherapy. When a psychiatric consultation or therapy is needed, the emphasis usually needs to be on assessing and improving the patient's coping resources and skills.

13

The Wisdom
of Hindsight

Six weeks after her breast lift and augmentation, Jackie summed up her experience:

> I don't think you can really appreciate what it's like until you've been through it. I thought I knew what to expect. I talked to my doctor at length. I talked to friends. I expected pain. And still, I didn't fully understand what I would experience. I'm happy with my results, but no one should underestimate the seriousness of this kind of operation. As my memory of the early recovery period fades, I may be able to say that I'd do it again. Right now, I'm not so sure.

Patients at all stages of recovery have provided their thoughts and advice for those who might be thinking about getting cosmetic surgery. Generally these comments fell into one of several areas, motivation and expectations for getting surgery, choosing a surgeon, deciding what to do, and coping with recovery.

Motivation and Expectations for Surgery

Anita, who got her first breast augmentation at 26, and six years later had it reversed, spoke of the need to think carefully before proceeding.

> At 26 I was just too young to know what I was doing. I thought I wanted to be sexy and appealing, but I didn't realize what it would be like to be made into a sex object. It was fun at first, but I found my augmented breasts to be cumbersome and restrictive. I couldn't do things I used to do, or wear things I used to wear. I wish I had been willing to do the work in therapy to better assess my motivations. My best advice is, know why you're doing it, and listen to your therapist.

Another patient said, "Be in a good place with yourself emotionally before having surgery. Otherwise you might be very disappointed." And another commented, "I waited a long time to get my nose done—I started thinking about it when I was in my teens. By the time it happened, it was a culmination of a long-awaited dream, mixed with anticipation of a change that had probably become greater, bigger than life, out of proportion to the reality."

Choosing a Surgeon

Robert had a face-lift and eyelid surgery and provided several tips about choosing and working with a surgeon. "Interview more than one plastic surgeon. The most expensive one is not necessarily the best. Be sure you have seen (or met) some of the patients who had the same surgery you are anticipating. Hopefully you'll see before-and-after pictures of these people. Show your surgeon pictures of features you like or dislike."

Another said, "Make sure you use a highly skilled, highly experienced (in their procedure), and highly recommended surgeon, and do *not* let cost be the sole determinant in choosing a surgeon." And again, "Check out the doctor's credentials and find at least one person who has been to him and talk to them in depth about their experience." And, "Do lots of research. Ask lots of people for referrals to surgeons. Pick the top three names that keep coming up. Then interview each of them. Pick the one that doesn't drink. I didn't want anyone with shaky hands operating on me."

Deciding What to Do

"Read all you can get on the subject."

One woman who had had a number of procedures done at once said, "Have surgery in small increments. Don't do too much at once. I think it would be easier emotionally and physically not to have a lot of trauma to deal with at once." Another said, "Everybody thinks nothing bad is going to happen to them. Be prepared for the worst and don't hesitate to call the doctor, but hope for the best."

Coping with Recovery

"Peas. Buy lots of frozen peas—more than you think you need." (This patient used frozen peas as cold compresses for her eyes during recovery from eyelid surgery.) A breast lift and augmentation patient said, "To discuss pain and to experience pain are two completely different things. I went into surgery fairly lightly, given how traumatic I discovered it was. I feel a loss of innocence, almost like losing my virginity." Paulette said, "I would ask to be asleep longer while the packing was in my nose, because that was the most difficult phase." Another said, "Lay there. Do nothing. Have all the help you can get during recovery."

Summary

Former patients summed up their thoughts and feelings after surgery:

"We are so lucky that we can decide whether to have cosmetic surgery. Some people don't have that option."

"I should have done it sooner! No pain, no gain."

"I'd do it again, but not the facial peel around the lips."

"Surgery was the last step in many that helped me to really know who and what I am and that I am worth it."

"I think most people feel better than they look afterwards."

Paulette said, "I'd do it again. The results were so great, and feeling that I no longer have to hide my profile makes me feel great. If someone were to say, 'Hey, you've got a great nose!' I'd say, 'Thank you. I do!' and really believe it."

Anita said, "I think breast augmentation is different from other cosmetic surgery. I had my nose done and I love it, but if I had it to do over again, I wouldn't have my boobs done."

The Australian woman whose difficult experience with breast augmentation was reported in Chapter 1 provided the following wisdom of hindsight:[1]

Maybe I'd want to see some photographs of other women before and after, or if I had read about other women and their problems it would have helped. Maybe I'd see a psychologist first and see whether counseling is an alternative. In retrospect I'd go away and think about it for a bit and ask around, or go to a medical library or get another opinion from another doctor or a nurse, not just my friend. I would like some instructions, maybe from the nurses, as to aftercare, what I should and shouldn't do. If I had any idea at all of what could happen I would have definitely waited another year because I remember thinking at the time, oh God, am I doing the right thing or not? But the doctor said he was going on holiday and if I wanted it done it would have to be in the next week. I think I rushed into it without enough forethought.

The vision of hindsight is said to be 20/20. It is much easier in retrospect to discern the course of action that would have been best. Most people who undergo cosmetic surgery are pleased with the results. Some must come to terms with the trade-offs between a perceived deficit in appearance and temporary or even lasting complications of surgery. The pain and trauma of the early recovery stage are almost always underestimated. Depending on the operation, cosmetic surgery impacts body image, sometimes significantly. Frequently, the reactions of others are unanticipated. These are among the many hazards along the road to a new, "possible self."

The decision to obtain cosmetic surgery is a very personal one, although it is influenced by many factors: personal beliefs and values, social taboos, judgments and reactions of friends and family, the pain of a perceived deficit, age and emotional maturity, and economic circumstances. It is crucial that those considering cosmetic surgery understand as fully as possible all that is entailed and carefully evaluate their motivation and expectations.

Epilogue

"I know exactly what you want!" said the sea witch. "It is stupid of you! But you shall have your way, for it is sure to bring you misfortune, my pretty Princess! You want to get rid of your fishtail and have, instead, two stumps that human beings use for walking, so that the young Prince may fall in love with you, and you may win him and an immortal soul! . . . I will make you a potion, and before sunrise you must swim ashore and sit on the beach and drink it. Then your tail will split in two and shrink into what human beings call legs. But I warn you it will hurt, as if a sharp sword were running through you. Everyone who sees you will say that you are the most beautiful child they have ever seen. You will keep your gracefulness, and no dancer will be able to move as lightly as you. But every step you take will be as painful as treading on a sharp knife. Are you willing to suffer all this?"

—From **The Little Mermaid**
by Hans Christian Andersen

Recently I ran into a former colleague whom I had not seen in 20 years. "Gee, you haven't changed a bit," he said, "You look great." He, on the other hand, looked every bit of 20 years older. Often I am asked if knowing what I know now, would I have cosmetic surgery again? I didn't have the answer to that question until I was well on the way to completion of this book. It is now four years since my surgery, and I finally know the answer. I would not do it the way I did four years ago—without careful consideration or a full understanding of what to expect. Weighing the costs and benefits would be very important. If I had had a fuller understanding at the time of my surgery, I think the emotional costs would have been less. Although I think my surgeon tried to inform me, I did not fully comprehend what he told me. The forces were already in motion. He *couldn't* tell me and I couldn't hear. Only now, after doing the research for this book, am I able to understand and appreciate what these forces were. Writing this book was a way of coming to terms with an experience that was painful and difficult. I want others to benefit from my experience. Still the question remains, would I do it again *knowing what I know now?*

Age discrimination is a reality, though often covert, and I have experienced it. Society has a variety of ways of invalidating older women. The face I see in the mirror now belies my actual age, and it better reflects how I feel inside. For that I'm grateful. I have accepted the skin discoloration, ear-lobe scars, scalp tightness, and changes in sensation that are all permanent reminders of my surgery in return for the improved appearance. I feel that my younger appearance gives me back some of the social and occupational advantage I had lost when I looked my age. I can now say, yes, I'm glad I had a face-lift, and I would do it again, but with the proviso that I would take care to be fully informed.

Appendix

American Board of Medical Specialties (ABMS)

The following are ABMS member specialty boards. Physicians and surgeons who are "board certified" by one or more of these boards have completed thousands of hours of training in the particular specialty the board addresses and have provided evidence of competency in the area for which certification is sought.

Members

American Board of Allergy & Immunology
American Board of Anesthesiology
American Board of Colon & Rectal Surgery
American Board of Dermatology
American Board of Emergency Medicine
American Board of Family Practice
American Board of Internal Medicine
American Board of Medical Genetics
American Board of Neurological Surgery
American Board of Nuclear Medicine
American Board of Obstetrics & Gynecology
American Board of Ophthalmology

American Board of Orthopedic Surgery
American Board of Otolaryngology
American Board of Pathology
American Board of Pediatrics
American Board of Physical Medicine and Rehabilitation
American Board of Plastic Surgery
American Board of Preventive Medicine
American Board of Psychiatry & Neurology
American Board of Radiology
American Board of Surgery
American Board of Thoracic Surgery
American Board of Urology

Reprinted with the permission of the American Board of Medical Specialties.

Self-Designated Boards

Self-designated boards are not recognized by ABMS as a member board. Although they purport to certify physicians and surgeons in the particular areas designated, requirements for training and competency vary widely and such boards have not subjected themselves to peer evaluation. Certification of competency from such organizations is probably meaningless.

The ABMS has been informed of the establishment of the following self-designated boards. They are called "American Board of _____" unless otherwise designated.

Abdominal Surgeons

Acupuncture Medicine

Addiction Medicine

Addictionology

Adolescent Psychiatry

Aesthetic Plastic Surgery

Alcoholism & Other Drug
    Dependencies (AMSAODD)

Algology (Chronic Pain)

Alternative Medicine

Ambulatory Anesthesia

Ambulatory Foot Surgery

Anesthesia

Arthroscopy (Board of North
America)

Arthroscopic Surgery

Bariatric Medicine

Bionic Psychology

Bloodless Medicine & Surgery

Cardiac Catheterization and
    Angiography

Chelation Therapy

Chemical Dependence

Clinical Chemistry

Clinical Ecology

Clinical Medicine and Surgery

Clinical Neurology

Clinical Neurophysiology

Clinical Neurosurgery

Clinical Nutrition

Clinical Orthopaedic Surgery

Clinical Pharmacology

Clinical Polysomnography

Clinical Psychiatry

Clinical Psychology

Clinical Toxicology

Cosmetic Plastic Surgery

Cosmetic Surgery

Council of Non-Board Certified Physicians

Critical Care of Medicine & Surgery

Dermalogy

Disability Evaluating Physicians

Electrodiagnostic Medicine

Electroencephalography

Electromyography and Electrodiagnosis

Environmental Medicine

Epidemiology (College)

Eye Surgery

Facial Cosmetic Surgery

Facial Plastic and Reconstructive Surgery

Family Practice, Certification in

Forensic Examiners

Forensic Psychiatry

Forensic Toxicology

Hand Surgery

Head, Facial & Neck Pain & TMJ Orthopedics

Health Physics

Homeopathic Physicians

Homeotherapeutics

Hypnotic Anesthesiology, National Board for

Independent Medical Examiners

Industrial Medicine & Surgery

Insurance Medicine

Int'l Cosmetic & Plastic Facial Reconstr. Stds.

Interventional Radiology

Laser Surgery

Law in Medicine

Longevity Medicine/Surgery

Malpractice Physicians

Maxillofacial Surgeons

Medical Accreditation (American Federation for)

Medical Hypnosis

Medical Laboratory Immunology

Medical-Legal Analysis of Medicine & Surgery

Medical Legal & Workers Comp.
Medicine & Surgery

Medical-Legal Consultants

Medical Management

Medical Microbiology

Medical Preventics (Academy)

Medical Psychotherapists

Medical Toxicology

Microbiology (Medical
Microbiology)

Military Medicine

Mohs Micrographic Surgery &
Cutaneous Oncology

Neuroimaging

Neurologic & Orthopedic Dental
Medicine & Surgery

Neurological & Orthopedic
Medicine

Neurological & Orthopedic
Surgery

Neurological Microsurgery

Neurology

Neuromuscular Thermography

Neuro-Orthop. Dental Medicine
& Surgery

Neuro-Orthop. Electrodiagnosis

Neuro-Orthop. Laser Surgery

Neuro-Orthop. Psychiatry

Neuro-Orthop. Thor.
Medicine/Surgery

Neurorehabilitation

Nutrition

Orthopedic Medicine

Orthopedic Microneurosurgery

Otorhinolaryngology

Pain Management (American
Academy of)

Pain Management Specialties

Pain Medicine

Percutaneous Diskectomy

Plastic Esthetic Surgeons

Prison Medicine

Professional Disability Consultants

Psychiatric Medicine

Psychiatry (American National Board
of)

Psychoanalysis (American Examining
Board in)

Psychological Medicine
(International)

Quality Assurance & Utilization
Review

Radiology and Medical Imaging

Rheumatologic Surgery

Rhematological & Reconstructive
Medicine

Ringside Medicine & Surgery

Skin Specialists

Sleep Medicine
(Polysomnography)

Spinal Cord Injury

Spinal Surgery

Sports Medicine

Sports Medicine/Surgery

Toxicology

Trauma Surgery

Traumatologic Medicine & Surgery

Tropical Medicine

Ultrasound Technology

Urological Surgery

Urologic Allied Health Professionals

Weight Reduction Medicine

Courtesy of the American Board of Medical Specialties.

Notes

Introduction

1. Shore 1992.
2. Reich 1969.
3. Goin, Burgoyne, Goin, and Staples 1980.
4. Johnston and Vogele 1993.

Chapter 1: Why Your Doctor *Can't* Tell You

1. Evans 1991, 19–20.
2. Evans 1991.
3. Baker, Kolin, and Barlett 1974.
4. McGregor and Greenberg 1972.
5. Leeb, Bowers, and Lynch 1976.
6. Goin, Burgoyne, and Goin 1976.
7. Hassar and Weintraub 1976.
8. Robinson and Merav 1976.
9. Evans 1991.

Chapter 2: Eye of the Beholder

1. Cash, Winstead, and Janda 1986.
2. Fitts, Gibson, Redding, and Deiter 1989.
3. Rosen, Reiter, and Orosan 1995.
4. Hay 1970.
5. Linn and Goldman 1949; Marcus 1984.
6. Kleck and Strenta 1980.
7. Frost and Peterson 1991.
8. Marcus 1984.

9. Beale, Lisper, and Palm 1980.
10. Harris 1989.
11. Rosen, Reiter, and Orosan 1995.
12. Cash 1995; Thompson 1990.
13. Fallon, Katzman, and Wooley 1994, 3–13.
14. Beale, Lisper, and Plam 1980; Edgerton, Meyer, and Jacobson 1961.
15. Beale, Lisper, and Palm 1980.
16. Wolf 1991, 14.
17. Carey 1989.
18. Rodin 1992, 26.
19. Freedman 1986.
20. Snyder, Tanke, and Berscheid 1977.
21. Eagly, Ashmore, Makhijani, and Longo 1991.
22. Kalick 1979.
23. Cash and Horton 1983.
24. Marcus 1984.
25. Reich 1969.

Chapter 3: In Pursuit of a Possible Self

1. Reich 1969.
2. Ohlsen, Ponten, and Hamberg 1979.
3. Landazuri 1992.
4. Breece and Nieberg 1986.
5. Frost and Peterson 1991.
6. Schweitzer 1989, 251.
7. Schlebusch 1989.
8. Mithers 1992, 83.
9. Macgregor 1989, 1.
10. Goin and Goin 1981, 122.
11. Meyer, Jacobson, Edgerton, and Canter 1960.
12. Druss 1973.
13. Edgerton and McClary 1958.
14. Webb, Slaughter, Meyer, and Edgerton 1965.
15. Baker and Smith 1939.
16. Hueston, Dennerstein, and Gotts 1985, 336.
17. Barsky 1944.
18. Hay 1970.
19. Hill and Silver 1950.
20. American Psychiatric Association 1994, 630.
21. Mohl 1984.
22. Macgregor 1974.
23. American Psychiatric Association 1994, xxi.
24. Undegraff and Menninger 1934.
25. Lasch 1979.
26. Edgerton, Meyer, and Jacobson 1961.
27. Reich 1969.
28. Webb, Slaughter, Meyer, and Edgerton 1965.
29. Goin and Goin 1981, 197–198.
30. Druss 1973.

31. Shipley, Donnell, and Bader 1977.
32. Beale, Lisper, and Palm 1980; Goin and Goin 1986; Hardy 1982; Hay 1970a.
33. Marcus 1984.
34. Macgregor 1967.
35. Macgregor 1989, 3.
36. Macgregor 1974.
37. Leppa 1990.
38. Freedman 1986.
39. Wolf 1991, 13.
40. Kegan 1982, 89.
41. Burk, Zelen, and Terino 1985.
42. Marcus and Nurius 1986.
43. Goin, Burgoyne, and Goin 1980.
44. Belfer, Mulliken, and Cochran 1979.
45. Schweitzer 1989, 251–252.
46. Wengle 1986, 439.

Chapter 4: "Cosmetic" Is Still Major Surgery

1. American Medical Association 1974.
2. Harris 1989.
3. Roach 1992.
4. Goin and Goin 1981.
5. Harris 1989.
6. Young, Brown, and Young 1991.
7. Bradbury, Hewison, and Timmons 1992.
8. Popp 1992.
9. Owsley 1983.
10. Scheck 1995.
11. Dillerud 1991.
12. Dillerud and Haheim 1993.
13. Drummond 1992.
14. Sun 1991.
15. Japenga 1993.
16. Rosenthal 1991.

Chapter 5: Who Seeks Surgery and Why

1. Japenga 1993.
2. Newman 1995.
3. Sabol 1991.
4. Stacey 1995.
5. Sabol 1991.
6. Drummond 1992.
7. Daniel 1991.
8. Goin 1988.
9. Daniel 1991.
10. ASPRS 1992.
11. Stal, Peterson, and Spira 1990.
12. Young, Brown, and Young 1991.
13. Blyth, Simmons, and Zakin 1985.

14. Bradbury, Hewison, and Timmons 1992
15. Stal, Peterson, and Spira 1990.
16. Bradbury, Hewison, and Timmons 1992.
17. Napoleon and Lewis 1990.
18. *The silicone scare* 1992.
19. Rosenthal 1991.
20. Grimes and Hunt 1993
21. Hawes and Bible 1990.
22. Gifford 1972.
23. Phillips 1991.
24. Jenike 1984.
25. Marks and Mishan 1988.
26. Hay 1970b.
27. Phillips 1991.
28. Brunswick 1928.
29. Hollander, Neville, Frenkel, Josephson, and Liebowitz 1992.
30. Andreasen and Bardach 1977; Fukuda 1977.
31. Andreasen and Bardach 1977.
32. Pertschuk 1991, 12.
33. Schweitzer 1989, 253.
34. Rubin 1994.
35. Morgan and Froning 1990.
36. Yates, Shisslak, Allender, and Wolman 1988.
37. McIntosh, Britt, and Bulik 1994.

Chapter 6: Okay, Schedule Me

1. Prochaska, DiClemente, and Norcross 1992.
2. Chrisler and Levy 1990.
3. Times Mirror 1990, 12.
4. Palcheff-Weimer, Concannon, Conn, and Puckett 1992.
5. Singer and Endreny 1987; Gunderson-Warner, Martinez, Martinez, Carey, Kochenour, and Emery 1990.
6. Robinson 1991.
7. *The silicone scare* 1992.
8. Palcheff-Wiemer et al. 1992.
9. ASPRS 1992.
10. Fraser 1990.
11. Robinson 1991.
12. Fraser 1990.
13. Johnston and Vogele 1993.
14. Mathews and Ridgeway 1984.
15. Hyatt 1986.

Chapter 7: What Have I Done?

1. Goldwyn 1991, 152.
2. Shore 1992.
3. Edgerton et al. 1960; Goin et al. 1980.
4. Goin 1978, 19–20.
5. Bradbury, Hewison, and Timmons 1992.

6. Bush 1987; Chapman 1956.
7. Barsky 1956; Edgerton, Jacobson, and Meyer 1960; Reich 1969.
8. Lindeman 1941.
9. Goin et al. 1980.
10. Edgerton, Meyer, and Jacobson 1961.
11. Harrell 1972.
12. Rosen 1950.
13. Polivy 1977.
14. Renneker and Cutler 1952; Maguire 1976.
15. Goin and Goin 1980.
16. Rosen and Shieff-Cahan 1993.
17. Tourkow 1974.
18. Goin and Goin 1981b.
19. Shore 1992.
20. National Institute of Mental Health 1987.
21. McGrath, Keita, Strickland, and Russo 1990.
22. Boyd and Weissman 1981, 1044.
23. Gilbert 1992, 62.
24. Gilbert 1992, 63.
25. Belsher and Costello 1988.
26. Farrant and Perez 1989; Whitlock and Siskind 1979.
27. Schulberg and Rush 1994.
28. Schulberg and Rush 1994.

Chapter 8: Mirror, Mirror . . . Who Is That?

1. Goin and Goin 1981b, 61.
2. Freud 1933.
3. Erikson 1956.
4. Fromm 1941.
5. Maslow 1954.
6. Rogers 1959.
7. Chein 1944.
8. Rosenberg 1979.
9. Goin and Goin 1986; Pruzinsky and Edgerton 1990, 217-235.
10. Pertschuk 1991, 16.
11. McIntosh, Britt, and Bulik 1994.
12. Edgerton, Langman, and Pruzinsky 1991, 604-605.
13. Goin and Goin 1981b, 163.
14. Beale, Lisper, and Palm 1980.
15. Zilbergeld 1978, 26-27.
16. Frost and Peterson 1991.
17. Goin 1978, 22.
18. Goin and Goin 1981, 205-206.
19. Thompson 1990.
20. Cash 1995.

Chapter 9: Your Nose Looks Okay to Me

1. Gullette 1991, 91, 127.
2. Barden 1991, 90, 126.

3. Goin and Goin 1986.
4. Wellisch, Jamison, and Pasnau 1978.
5. Goldwyn 1991.

Chapter 10: I Like How I Look, But ...

1. Reich 1975.
2. Beller and Wagner 1980; Schultz-Coulon 1977.
3. Wengle 1986a.
4. Beller and Wagner 1980.
5. Landazuri 1992.
6. Putterman 1990.
7. ASPRS 1992a.
8. Dillerud 1991; Illouz and deVillers 1989.
9. Dillerud 1991.
10. Dillerud and Haheim 1993.
11. Goin, Burgoyne, Goin, and Staples 1980.
12. Edgerton, Webb, Slaughter, and Meyer 1964.
13. Klabunde and Falces 1964.
14. Goin and Rees 1991.
15. Schultz-Coulon 1977.
16. Marcus 1984.
17. Strombeck 1964; Pers, Nielsen, and Gerner 1986.
18. Serletti, Reading, Caldwell, and Wray 1992.
19. Leist, Masson, and Erich 1977.
20. Linn and Goldman 1949.
21. Goin and Goin 1986, 99.
22. Schweitzer 1989, 251.
23. Edgerton, Jacobson, and Meyer, 1960.
24. Wright and Wright 1975.
25. Marcus 1984.
26. Goin and Goin 1979.
27. Edgerton, Webb, Slaughter, and Meyer 1964; Webb, Slaughter, Meyer, and Edgerton 1965.
28. Goin, Burgoyne, Goin, and Staples 1980.
29. Edgerton and McClary 1958.
30. Burning 1992.
31. Druss 1973.
32. Wengle 1986b.

Chapter 11: I Paid Good Money for This?

1. Goin and Goin 1986.
2. Goin and Goin 1986.
3. Knorr 1972.
4. Hinderer 1978.
5. Kron 1994.
6. Wright 1986.
7. Leppa 1990.
8. Asken 1975.
9. Druss, Symonds, and Crickelair 1971.

10. Goin and Goin 1986.
11. Schweitzer and Hirschfeld 1984.
12. Goin and Goin, 1981b, p. 98.
13. Scheer 1992.
14. Robinson 1991.
15. Robinson 1991.
16. Robinson 1991.
17. Macgregor 1981.

Chapter 12: Surgery or Therapy?

1. Greer 1984.
2. Wengle 1986b, 490.
3. Stone and Porter 1995.
4. Lazarus 1986.
5. Schwartz, Lerman, Miller, Daly, and Masny 1995.
6. Lerman and Schwartz 1993.
7. Schwartz, Lerman, Miller, Daly, and Masny 1995.
8. Griffith and Griffith 1994.

Chapter 13: The Wisdom of Hindsight

1. Evans 1991, 27.

Bibliography

American Medical Association. (1974). *Proceedings of the house of delegates: Adoption of resolution 78 (A-74).* 28th Clinical Convention, Portland, OR, December 1–4.

American Psychiatric Association. (1994). *Diagnostic and statistical manual of mental disorders,* (4th ed.). Washington, DC: American Psychiatric Association.

American Society of Plastic and Reconstructive Surgeons. (1992a). *Results of telephone survey of female consumers.* Arlington Heights, IL: American Society of Plastic and Reconstructive Surgeons.

American Society of Plastic and Reconstructive Surgeons. (1992b). *1992 Statistics.* Arlington Heights, IL: American Society of Plastic and Reconstructive Surgeons.

Andreasen, N. C., and Bardach, J. (1977). Dysmorphophobia: Symptom or disease? *American Journal of Psychiatry, 134,* 673–676.

Asken, M. J. (1975). Psychoemotional aspects of mastectomy: A review of recent literature. *American Journal of Psychiatry, 132,* 56–59.

Baker, J. L., Kolin, I. S., and Bartlett, E. S. (1974). Psychosexual dynamics of patients undergoing mammary augmentation. *Plastic and Reconstructive Surgery, 53,* 652–659.

Baker, W. Y., and Smith, L. H. (1939). Facial disfigurement and personality. *Journal of the American Medical Association, 112,* 301–309.

Barden, C. I. (1991). Facelift: Pro. *Lear's,* March, 90, 126.

Barsky, A. J. (1944). Psychology of the patient undergoing plastic surgery. *American Journal of Surgery, 65,* 238–242.

Barsky, A. J. (1956). Psychosomatic medicine and plastic surgery. In A. J. Cantor and A. N. Foxe (Eds.), *Psychosomatic aspects of surgery.* New York: Grune and Stratton.

Beale, S., Lisper, H. O., and Palm, B. (1980). A psychological study of patients seeking augmentation mammaplasty. *British Journal of Psychiatry, 136,* 133–138.

Belfer, M. L., Mulliken, J. B., and Cochran, T. C. (1979). Cosmetic surgery as an antecedent of life change. *American Journal of Psychiatry, 136,* 199–201.

Beller, F. K., and Wagner, H. (1980). Ergebnisse nach reduktionsplastiken der weiblihen brust. *Geburtsh Frauenheilkd, 40,* 112.

Belsher, G., and Costello, C. G. (1988). Relapse from recovery from unipolar depression: A critical review. *Psychological Bulletin, 104,* 84–86.

Berscheid, E. (1981). An overview of the psychological effects of physical attractiveness. In G. W. Lucker, K. A. Ribbens, and J. A. McNamara (Eds.), *Psychological aspects of facial form* (Craniofacial growth series). Center for Human Growth and Development, University of Michigan, 1.

Berscheid, E., and Gangstead, S. (1982). The social implications of facial physical attractiveness. *Clinical Plastic Surgery, 9,* 289–293.

Blyth, D. A., Simmons, R. G., and Zakin, D. F. (1985). Satisfaction with body image for early adolescent females: The impact of pubertal timing within different school environments. *Journal of Youth and Adolescence, 14,* 207–225.

Boyd, J. H., and Weissman, M. M. (1981). Epidemiology of affective disorders. *Archives of General Psychiatry, 38,* 1039–1046.

Bradbury, E. T., Hewison, J., and Timmons, M. J. (1992). Psychological and social outcome of prominent ear correction in children. *British Journal of Plastic Surgery, 45,* 97–100.

Breece, G. L., and Nieberg, L. G. (1986). Motivations for adult orthodontic treatment. *Journal of Clinical Orthodontia, 20,* 166–171.

Bronheim, H., Strain, J. J., and Biller, H. F. (1991). Psychiatric aspects of head and neck surgery, Part II: Body image and psychiatric intervention. *General Hospital Psychiatry, 13,* 225–232.

Bruning, N. (1992). *Breast implants: Everything you need to know.* Alameda, CA: Hunter House.

Brunswick, R. M. (1928). A supplement to Freud's "History of an infantile neurosis." *International Journal of Psychoanalysis, 9,* 439–476.

Burk, J., Zelen, S. L., and Terino, E. O. (1985). More than skin deep: A self-consistency approach to the psychology of cosmetic surgery. *Plastic and Reconstructive Surgery, 76,* 270–277.

Bush, J. P. (1987). Pain in children: A review of the literature and a developmental perspective. *Psychology and Health, 1,* 215–221.

Carey, J. S. (1989). Kant and the cosmetic surgeon. *Journal of the Florida Medical Association, 76,* 637–643.

Cash, T. F. (1995). *What do you see when you look in the mirror? Helping yourself to a positive body image.* New York: Bantam.

Cash, T. F., and Horton, C. E. (1983). Aesthetic surgery: Effects of rhinoplasty on the social perception of patients by others. *Plastic and Reconstructive Surgery, 72,* 543–548.

Cash, T. F., and Pruzinsky, T. (1990). *Body images: Development, deviance, and change.* New York: Guilford Press.

Cash, T. F., Winstead, B. A., and Janda, L. H. (1986). The great American shape-up: Body image survey report. *Psychology Today,* April, 30–34, 36–37.

Chapman, A. H., Loeb, D. G., and Gibbons, M. J. (1956). Psychiatric aspects of hospitalizing children. *Archives of Pediatrics, 73,* 7–11.

Chein, I. (1944). The awareness of self and the structure of the ego. *Psychological Review, 51,* 304–314.

Chrisler, J., and Levy, K. (1990). The media construct a menstrual monster: A content analysis of the PMS articles in the popular press. *Women and Health, 16,* 89.

Daniel, R. K. (1991). Rhinoplasty and the male patient. *Clinics in Plastic Surgery, 18,* 751–761.

Dillerud, E. (1991). Suction lipoplasty: A report on complications, undesired results, and patient satisfaction based on 3511 procedures. *Plastic and Reconstructive Surgery, 88,* 239–248.

Dillerud, E., and Haheim, L. L. (1993). Long-term results of blunt section lipectomy assessed by patient questionnaire survey. *Plastic and Reconstructive Surgery, 92,* 35–42.

Drummond, M. (1992). Homme improvements. *New Woman,* May, 51–53.

Druss, R. G. (1973). Changes in the body image following augmentation breast surgery. *Journal of Psychoanalytic Psychotherapy, 2,* 248–256.

Druss, R. G., Symonds, F. C., and Crickelair, G. L. (1971). The problem of somatic delusions in patients seeking cosmetic surgery. *Plastic and Reconstructive Surgery, 46,* 246–250.

Eagly, A. H., Ashmore, R. D., Makhijani, M. G., and Longo, L. C. (1991). What is beautiful is good, but . . . : A meta-analytic review of research on the physical attractiveness stereotype. *Psychological Bulletin, 110,* 109–128.

Edgerton, M. T., Jacobson, W. E., and Meyer. E. (1960). Surgical psychiatric study of patients seeking plastic (cosmetic) surgery: Ninety-eight consecutive patients with minimal deformity. *British Journal of Plastic Surgery, 13,* 136–145.

Edgerton, M. T., Langman, M. W., and Pruzinsky, T. (1991). Plastic surgery and psychotherapy in the treatment of 100 psychologically disturbed patients. *Plastic and Reconstructive Surgery, 88,* 594–608.

Edgerton, M. T., and McClary, A. R. (1958). Augmentation mammaplasty, psychiatric implications and surgical indications. *Plastic and Reconstructive Surgery, 21,* 279–284.

Edgerton, M. T., Meyer, E., and Jacobson, W. E. (1961). Augmentation mammaplasty: II. Further surgical and psychiatric evaluations. *Plastic and Reconstructive Surgery, 27,* 279–305.

Edgerton, M. T., Webb, W. L., Slaughter, R., and Meyer, E., (1964). Surgical results and psychosocial changes following rhytidectomy. *Plastic and Reconstructive Surgery, 33,* 503–521.

Erikson, E. (1956). The problem of ego identity. *Journal of the American Psychoanalytic Association, 4,* 56–121.

Evans, M. (1991). Augmentation mammaplasty: Neither simple nor safe. *The Australian Journal of Advanced Nursing, 8,* 19–28.

Fallon, P., Katzman, M. A., and Wooley, S. C. (1994). *Feminist perspectives on eating disorders.* New York: Guilford Press.

Farrant, J., and Perez, M. (1989). Immunity and depression. In J. G. Howells (Ed.), *Modern perspectives in the psychiatry of the affective disorders: Modern perspectives in psychiatry, Vol. 13.* New York: Brunner/Mazel.

Fisher, S., and Cleveland, S. E. (1958). *Body image and personality.* Princeton, NJ: D. Van Nostrand.

Fitts, S. N., Gibson, P., Redding, C. A., and Deiter, P. J. (1989). Body dysmorphic disorder: Implications for its validity as a DSM-III-R clinical syndrome. *Psychological Reports, 64,* 655–658.

Fraser, L. (1990). The cosmetic surgery hoax. *Glamour,* February, 184, 220–224.

Freedman, R. J. (1986). *Beauty bound.* New York: D. C. Heath.

Freud, S. (1923). *The ego and the id. Standard edition XIX.* London: Hogorth Press, 26.

Freud, S. (1933). *A new series of introductory lectures on psycho-analysis.* (Translated by W. J. H. Sprott.) New York: W. W. Norton.

Fromm, E. (1941). *Escape from Freedom.* New York: Holt.

Frost, V., and Peterson, G. (1991). Psychological aspects of orthognathic surgery: How people respond to facial change. *Oral Surgery, Oral Medicine, Oral Pathology, 71,* 538–542.

Fukuda, O. (1977). Statistical analysis of dysmorphophobia in an out-patient clinic. *Japanese Journal of Plastic & Reconstructive Surgery, 20,* i569–i577.

Gifford, S. (1972). Cosmetic surgery and personality change: A review and some clinical observations. In R. M. Goldwyn (Ed.), *The unfavorable result in plastic surgery.* Boston: Little, Brown.

Gilbert, P. (1992). *Depression: The evolution of powerlessness.* New York: Guilford Press.

Goin, J. M., and Goin, M. K. (1981a). Midlife reactions to mastectomy and subsequent breast reconstruction. *Archives of General Psychiatry, 38.*

Goin, J. M., and Goin, M. K. (1981b). *Changing the body: Psychological effects of plastic surgery.* Baltimore: William and Wilkens.

Goin, M. K. (1978). Psychiatric considerations. In E. H. Courtiss, (Ed.) *Aesthetic surgery: Trouble—how to avoid it and how to treat it.* St. Louis, MO: Mosby. 17–24.

Goin, M. K. (1988). Psychological understanding and management of rhinoplasty patients. *Clinical Plastic Surgery, 4,* 3–9.

Goin, M. K., Burgoyne, R. W., and Goin, J. M. (1976). Face-lift operation: The patient's secret motivations and reactions to "informed consent." *Plastic and Reconstructive Surgery, 58,* 273–279.

Goin, M. K., Burgoyne, R. W., Goin J. M., and Staples, F. R. (1980). A prospective psychological study of 50 female face-lift patients. *Plastic and Reconstructive Surgery, 65,* 436–442.

Goin, M. K., and Goin, J. M. (1979, October). *Psychoanalytic perspectives of rhinoplasty.* Presented to the American Society of Plastic and Reconstructive Surgeons, San Francisco.

Goin, M. K., and Goin, J. M. (1986). Psychological effects of aesthetic facial surgery. *Advances in Psychosomatic Medicine, 15,* 84–108.

Goin, M. K., and Rees, T. D. (1991). A prospective study of patients' psychological reactions to rhinoplasty. *Annals of Plastic Surgery, 27,* 210–215.

Goldwyn, R. M. (1991). *The patient and the plastic surgeon,* 2nd. ed. Boston: Little, Brown.

Gorman, A. (1993). Surgeons explore ethnic beauty. *Plastic Surgery News,* American Society of Plastic and Reconstructive Surgeons, April, 1, 15.

Greer, D. M. (1984). Psychiatric consultation in plastic surgery: The surgeon's perspective. *Psychosomatics, 25,* 470, 472–474.

Griffith, J. L., and Griffith, M. E. (1994). *The body speaks: Therapeutic dialogues for mind-body problems.* New York: Basic Books.

Grimes, P. E., and Hunt, S. G. (1993). Considerations for cosmetic surgery in the black population. *Clinics in Plastic Surgery, 20,* 27–34.

Groenman, N. H., and Sauer, H. C. (1983). Personality characteristics of the cosmetic surgical insatiable patient. *Psychotherapy and Psychosomatics, 40,* 241–245.

Gullette, M. M. (1991). Facelift: Con. *Lear's,* March, 91, 127.

Gunderson-Warner, S., Martinez, L. P., Martinez, I. P., Carey, J. C., Kochenour, N. K., and Emery, M. G. (1990). Critical review of articles regarding pregnancy exposures in popular magazines. *Teratology, 42,* 469–476.

Hardy, G. E. (1982). Body image disturbance is dysmorphophobia. *British Journal of Psychiatry, 141,* 181–185.

Harris, D. L. (1989). Cosmetic surgery. *Annals of the Royal College of Surgeons of England, 71,* 195–199.

Harrell, H. C. (1972). To lose a breast. *American Journal of Nursing, 72,* 676–677.

Hassar, M., and Weintraub, M. (1976). Uninformed consent and the wealthy volunteer: An analysis of patient volunteers in a clinical trial of a new anti-inflammatory drug. *Clinical Pharmacological Therapy, 20,* 379–386.

Hawes, M. J., and Bible, H. H. (1990). The paranoid patient: Surgeon beware! *Ophthalmic Plastic and Reconstructive Surgery, 6,* 225–227.

Hay, G. G. (1970a). Psychiatric aspects of cosmetic nasal operations. *British Journal of Psychiatry, 116,* 85–90.

Hay, G. G. (1970b). Dysmorphophobia. *British Journal of Psychiatry, 116,* 399–406.

Hetter, G. P. (1979). Satisfactions and dissatisfactions of patients with augmentation mammaplasty. *Plastic and Reconstructive Surgery, 64,* 151–158.

Hill, G., and Silver, A. G. (1950). Psychodynamic and aesthetic motivations for plastic surgery. *Psychosomatic Medicine, 12,* 345–351.

Hinderer, U. T. (1978). Dr. Vazquez Anon's last lesson. *Aesthetic Plastic Surgery, 2,* 375–382.

Hollander, E., Neville, D., Frenkel, M., Josephson, S., and Liebowitz, M. R. (1992). Body dysmorphic disorder: Diagnostic issues and related disorders. *Psychosomatics, 33,* 156–165.

Hueston, J., Dennerstein, L., and Gotts, G. (1985). Psychological aspects of cosmetic surgery. *Journal of Psychosomatic Obstetrics and Gynecology, 4,* 335–346.

Hyatt, R. (1986). Psychological effects of surgery and hospitalization. *USA Today,* November, 90–92.

Illouz, Y. G., and deVillers, Y. T. (1989). *Body sculpturing by lipoplasty.* New York: Churchill-Livingstone.

Jackson, L. A. (1992). *Physical appearance and gender: Sociobiological and sociocultural perspectives.* Albany: State University of New York Press.

Japenga, A. (1993). Face lift city. *Health,* March/April, 47–48, 51–52, 55.

Jenike, M. A. (1984). A case report of successful treatment of dysmorphophobia with tranylcypromine. *American Journal of Psychiatry, 141,* 1463–1464.

Johnston, M., and Vogele, C. (1993). Benefits of psychological preparation for surgery: A meta-analysis. *Annals of Behavioral Medicine, 15,* 245–256.

Kalick, S. M. (1979). Aesthetic surgery: How it affects the way patients are perceived by others. *Annals of Plastic Surgery, 2,* 128–132.

Kegan, R. (1982). *The evolving self: Problem and process in human development.* Cambridge, MA: Harvard University Press.

Klabunde, E. H., and Falces, E. (1964). Incidence of complications in cosmetic rhinoplasties. *Plastic and Reconstructive Surgery, 34,* 192–197.

Kleck, R. E., and Strenta, A. (1980). Perceptions of the impact of negatively valued physical characteristics on social interaction. *Journal of Personality and Social Psychology, 39,* 861–868.

Knorr, N. J. (1972). Feminine loss of identity in rhinoplasty. *Archives of Otolaryngology, 96,* 11–15.

Knorr, N. J., Edgerton, M. T., and Hoopes, J. E. (1967). The "insatiable" cosmetic surgery patient. *Plastic and Reconstructive Surgery, 40,* 285–289.

Kron, J. (1994). Appointment with death. *Allure,* February, 102–105, 147.

Landazuri, H. (1992). Plastic surgery and psychology: Study of 1000 consecutive cases. *Plastic Surgery, 1,* 17–19.

Lasch, C. (1979). *The culture of narcissism.* New York: Warner Books.

Lazarus, R. S. (1986). *Psychological stress and the coping process.* New York: McGraw-Hill.

Leeb, D., Bowers, D. G., Jr., and Lynch, J. B. (1976). Observations on the myth of informed consent. *Plastic and Reconstructive Surgery, 58,* 280–282.

Leist, S. D., Masson, J. K., and Erich, J. B. (1977). A review of 324 rhytidetomies, emphasizing complications and patient dissatisfaction. *Plastic and Reconstructive Surgery, 59,* 525–529.

Leppa, C. J. (1990). Cosmetic surgery and the motivation for health and beauty. *Nursing Forum, 25,* 25–31.

Lerman, C., and Schwartz, M. D. (1993). Adherence and psychological adjustment among women at high risk for breast cancer. *Breast Cancer Research and Treatment, 28,* 145–155.

Lindemann, E. (1941). Observations on psychiatric sequelae to surgical operations in women. *American Journal of Psychiatry, 98,* 132–138.

Linn, L., and Goldman, I. (1949). Psychiatric observations concerning rhinoplasty. *Psychosomatic Medicine, 11,* 307–314.

Macgregor, F. C. (1967). Social and cultural components in the motivations of persons seeking plastic surgery of the nose. *Journal of Health and Social Behavior, 8,* 125–131.

Macgregor, F. C. (1974). *Transformation and identity: The face and plastic surgery.* New York: Quadrangle/New York Times Book Company.

Macgregor, F. C. (1981). Patient dissatisfaction with results of technically satisfactory surgery. *Aesthetic Plastic Surgery, 5,* 27–32.

Macgregor, F. C. (1989). Social, psychological and cultural dimensions of cosmetic and reconstructive plastic surgery. *Aesthetic Plastic Surgery, 13,* 1–8.

Maguire, P. (1976). The psychological and social sequelae of mastectomy. In J. G. Howells (Ed.), *Modern perspectives in the psychiatric aspects of surgery.* New York: Brunner/Mazel.

Marcus, P. (1984). Psychological aspects of cosmetic rhinoplasty. *British Journal of Plastic Surgery, 37,* 313–318.

Marks, I., and Mishan, J. (1988). Dysmorphophobic avoidance with disturbed bodily perception: A pilot study of exposure therapy. *British Journal of Psychiatry, 152,* 674–678.

Markus, H., and Nurius, P. (1986). Possible selves. *American Psychologist, 41,* 954–969.

Maslow, A. H. (1954). *Motivation and personality.* New York: Harper.

Mathews, A., and Ridgeway, V. (1984). Psychological preparation for surgery. In Steptoe, A., and Mathews, A. (Eds.), *Health care and human behaviour.* London: Academic Press, 231–259.

McGregor, M. W., and Greenberg, R. L. (1972). In R. M. Goldwyn (Ed.), *The unfavorable result in plastic surgery.* Boston: Little, Brown.

McGrath, E., Keita, G. P., Strickland, B., and Russo, N. F. (Eds.). (1990). *Women and depression: Risk factors and treatment issues.* Washington, DC: American Psychological Association.

McIntosh, V. V., Britt, E., and Bulik, C. M. (1994). Cosmetic breast augmentation and eating disorders. *New Zealand Medical Journal, 107,* 151–152.

McKinney, P., and Cook, J. Q. (1981). A critical evaluation of 200 rhinoplasties. *Annals of Plastic Surgery, 24,* 357–363.

Meyer, E., Jacobson, W. E., Edgerton, M. T., and Canter, A. (1960). Motivational patterns in patients seeking elective plastic surgery: I. Women who seek rhinoplasty. *Psychosomatic Medicine, 22,* 193–199.

Mithers, C. L. (1992). Why women want man-made breasts. *McCall's*, April, 83.

Mohl, P. C. (1984). Psychiatric consultation in plastic surgery: The psychiatrist's perspective. *Psychosomatics, 25*, 471, 474–476.

Morgan, E., and Froning, M. L. (1990). Child sexual abuse sequelae and body-image surgery. *Plastic and Reconstructive Surgery, 86*, 475–478.

Napoleon, A., and Lewis, C. M. (1989). Psychological considerations in lipoplasty: The problematic or "special care" patient. *Annals of Plastic Surgery, 23*, 430–432.

Napoleon, A., and Lewis, C. M. (1990). Psychological considerations in the elderly cosmetic surgery candidate. *Annals of Plastic Surgery, 24*, 165–169.

National Institute of Mental Health. (1987). *National lesbian health care survey.* Washington, DC: U.S. Government Printing Office.

Newman, J. (1995). Scalpelmania! *Elle*, March, 256, 258, 260.

Ohlsen, L., Ponten, B., and Hamberg, G. (1979). Augmentation mammaplasty: A surgical and psychiatric evaluation of the results. *Annals of Plastic Surgery, 2*, 42–52.

Owsley, J. Q. (1983). SMAS-platysma face lift. *Plastic and Reconstructive Surgery, 71*, 573–576.

Palcheff-Wiemer, M., Concannon, M. J., Conn, V. S., and Puckett, C. L. (1992). The impact of the media on women with breast implants. *Plastic and Reconstructive Surgery, 92*, 779–785.

Pers, M., Nielsen, I., and Gerner, N. (1986). Results following reduction mammoplasty as evaluated by the patient. *Annals of Plastic and Reconstructive Surgery, 17*, 449–455.

Pertschuk, M. (1991). Psychosocial considerations in interface surgery. *Clinics in Plastic Surgery, 18*, 11–18.

Phillips, K. A. (1991). Body dysmorphic disorder: The distress of imagined ugliness. *American Journal of Psychiatry, 148*, 1138–1149.

Polivy, J. (1977). Psychological effects of mastectomy on a woman's feminine self-concept. *Journal of Nervous Mental Disorders, 164*, 77–87.

Popp, J. C. (1992). Complications of blepharoplasty and their management. *Journal of Dermatological Surgery and Oncology, 18*, 1122–1126.

President's Commission for the Study of Ethical Problems in Medicine and Biomedical and Behavioral Research: Making health care decisions. (1982). *The ethical and legal implications of informed consent in the patient-practitioner relationship: Volume one: Report.* Washington, DC: U.S. Government Printing Office.

Prochaska, J. O., DiClemente, C. C., and Norcross, J. C. (1992). In search of how people change. *American Psychologist, 47*, 1102–1114.

Pruzinsky, T. (1993). Psychological factors in cosmetic plastic surgery: Recent developments in patient care. *Plastic Surgical Nursing, 13,* 64–119.

Pruzinsky, T., and Edgerton, M. T. (1990). Body-image change in cosmetic plastic surgery. In Cash, T. F., and Pruzinsky, T. (Eds.), *Body images: Development, deviance, and change.* New York: Guilford Press, 217–236.

Putterman, A. M. (1990). Patient satisfaction in oculoplastic surgery. *Ophthalmic Surgery, 21,* 15–21.

Renneker, R., and Cutler, M. (1952). Psychological problems of adjustment to cancer of the breast. *Journal of the American Medical Association, 148,* 833–839.

Reich, J. (1969). The surgery of appearance: Psychological and related aspects. *Medical Journal of Australia, 2,* 5–14.

Reich, J. (1975). Factors influencing patient satisfaction with the results of aesthetic plastic surgery. *Plastic and Reconstructive Surgery, 55,* 5–10.

Roach, M. (1992). The latest lift. *Vogue,* October.

Robinson, D. (1991). The truth about cosmetic surgery. *Reader's Digest,* February, 75–80.

Robinson, G., and Merav, A. (1976). Informed consent: Recall by patients tested post-operatively. *Annals of Thoractic Surgery, 22,* 209–212.

Rodin, J. (1992). *Body traps: Breaking the binds that keep you from feeling good about your body.* New York: William Morrow.

Rogers, C. (1959). A theory of therapy, personality, and interpersonal relationships as developed in the client centered framework. In S. Koch (Ed.), *Psychology: A study of science, Vol. 3: Formulations of the person and the social context.* New York: McGraw-Hill.

Rosen, J. C., Reiter, J., and Orosan, P. (1995). Cognitive-behavioral body image therapy for body dysmorphic disorder. *Journal of Consulting and Clinical Psychology, 63,* 263–269.

Rosen, M., and Shieff-Cahan, V. (1993). Now I can be free. *People Magazine, 16,* April 26, 82–84, 87.

Rosen, V. H. (1950). The role of denial in acute postoperative affective reactions following removal of a body part. *Psychosomatic Medicine, 12,* 356–361.

Rosenberg, M. (1979). *Conceiving the self.* New York: Basic Books.

Rosenthal, E. (1991). Ethnic ideals: Rethinking plastic surgery. *New York Times,* September 25.

Rubin, S. (1994). Her face is a work of art. *San Francisco Chronicle,* February 4, C1, C16.

Sabol, B. (1991). Nip and tuck: The plastic-surgery fix is America's new addiction. *Self*, March, 102.

Scheck, A. (1995, January 24). Several new cosmetic surgeries for men. *Investor's Business Daily*, 1-2.

Scheer, R., (with O'Connor, K.) (1992). *The cosmetic surgery revolution.* Los Angeles: Summit Pines Press.

Schein, J. (1992). Cosmetic surgery: A nip and a tuck. *Consumer's Research,* September, 30–34.

Schilder, P. (1950). *The image and appearance of the human body.* New York: International University Press.

Schlebusch, L. (1989). Negative bodily experience and prevalence of depression in patients who request augmentation mammoplasty. *South African Medical Journal, 75,* 323–326.

Schulberg, H. C., and Rush, A. J. (1994). Clinical practice guidelines for managing major depression in primary care practice. *American Psychologist, 49,* 34–41.

Schultz-Coulon, H. J. (1977). Rhinoplastik—ein uberwiegend aesthetischer oder funktioneller Eingriff? *Laryngol Rhinol, 56,* 233.

Schwartz, M. D., Lerman, C., Miller, S. M., Daly, M., and Masny, A. (1995). Coping disposition, perceived risk, and psychological distress among women at increased risk for ovarian cancer. *Health Psychology, 14,* 232–235.

Schweitzer, I. (1989). The psychiatric assessment of the patient requesting facial surgery. *Australian and New Zealand Journal of Psychiatry, 23,* 249–254.

Schweitzer, I., and Hirschfeld, J. J. (1984). Postrhytidectomy psychosis: A rare complication. *Plastic and Reconstructive Surgery, 74,* 419–421.

Serletti, J. M., Reading, G., Caldwell, E., and Wray, R. C. (1992). Long-term patient satisfaction following reduction mammoplasty. *Annals of Plastic Surgery, 28,* 363–365.

Shipley, R. H., Donnell, J. M., and Bader, K. F. (1977). Personality characteristics of women seeking breast augmentation. *Plastic and Reconstructive Surgery, 60,* 369–379.

Shore, S. C. (1992). An exploratory study of postoperative trauma and depression among cosmetic surgery recipients. (Doctoral dissertation, The Union Institute). *Dissertation Abstracts International, 53,* 1102-B.

Singer, E., and Endreny, P. (1987). Reporting hazards: Their benefits and costs. *Journal of Communication, 37,* 10.

Snyder, M., Tanke, E., and Berscheid, E. (1977). Social perception and interpersonal behavior: On the self-fulfilling nature of social stereotypes. *Journal of Personality and Social Psychology, 35,* 656–666.

Stacey, M. (1995). I am woman, lift my breasts. *Elle*, March, 264.

Stal, S., Peterson, R., and Spira, M. (1990). Aesthetic considerations and the pediatric population. *Clinics in Plastic Surgery, 17*, 133–149.

Stone, A. A., and Porter, L. S. (1995). Psychological coping: Its importance for treating medical problems. *Mind/Body Medicine, 1*, 46–54.

Strombeck, J. O. (1964). Macromastia in women and its surgical treatment. *Acta Chir Scandinavia, 341 (Supplement)*, 1–128.

Sun, L. H. (1991). A growth industry in China: Penile augmentation. *Washington Post*, November 17.

The silicone scare. (1992). *First for Women*, June 8, 16–17.

Thomas, C. S. (1990). Stress and facial appearance. *Stress Medicine, 6*, 299–304.

Thompson, J. K. (1990). *Body image disturbance: Assessment and treatment*. New York: Pergamon Press.

Tiemersma, D. (1989). *Body schema and body image: An interdisciplinary and philosophical study*. Amsterdam/Lisse: Swets and Zeitlinger.

Times Mirror Center of the People and the Press. (1990). The American media: Who reads, who watches, who listens, who cares. *Advertising Age, 61*, July 30, 12.

Tourkow, L. P. (1974). Psychic consequences of loss and replacement of body parts. *Journal of the American Psychoanalytic Association, 22*, 170–181.

Undergraff, H. L., and Menninger, K. A. (1934). Some psychoanalytic aspects of plastic surgery. *American Journal of Plastic Surgery, 25*, 554–565.

Webb, W. L., Slaughter, R., Meyer, E., and Edgerton, M. T. (1965). Mechanisms of psychosocial adjustment in patients seeking "face-lift" operation. *Psychosomatic Medicine, 27*, 183–192.

Wengle, H. P. (1986a). The psychology of cosmetic surgery: A critical overview of the literature 1960–1982—Part I, *Annals of Plastic Surgery, 16*, 435–443.

Wengle, H. P. (1986b). The psychology of cosmetic surgery: Old problems in patient selection seen in a new way—Part II, *Annals of Plastic Surgery, 16*, 487–492.

Wellisch, D. K., Jamison, K. R., and Pasnau, R. O. (1978). Psychosocial aspects of mastectomy: II. The man's perspective. *American Journal of Psychiatry, 136*, 543–546.

Whitlock, F. A., and Siskind, M. (1979). Depression and cancer: A follow-up study. *Psychological Medicine, 9*, 747–752.

Wolf, N. (1991). *The beauty myth*. New York: Anchor Books.

Wright, M. R. (1980). Self perception of the elective surgeon and some patient perception correlates. *Archives of Otolaryngology, 106*, 460.

Wright, M. R. (1986). Surgical addiction: A complication of modern surgery? *Archives of Otolaryngology and Head and Neck Surgery, 112*, 870–872.

Wright, M. R. and Wright, W. K. (1975). A psychological study of patients undergoing cosmetic surgery. *Archives of Otolaryngology, 101*, 125–131.

Yates, A., Shisslak, C. M., Allender, J. R., and Wolman, W. (1988). Plastic surgery and the bulimic patient. *International Journal of Eating Disorders, 7*, 557–560.

Young, V. L., Brown, D. M., and Young, A. E. (1991). Gynecomastia. *Missouri Medicine, 88*, 153–158.

Zilbergeld, B. (1978). *Male sexuality.* New York: Bantam Books.

Other New Harbinger Self-Help Titles